Botox And Fillers

Editors
EVAN BUSBY
TIRBOD FATTAHI

ATLAS OF THE ORAL AND MAXILLOFACIAL SURGERY CLINICS OF NORTH AMERICA

www.oralmaxsurgeryatlas.theclinics.com

Consulting Editor
RUI P. FERNANDES

March 2024 • Volume 32 • Number 1

ELSEVIER

1600 John F. Kennedy Boulevard • Suite 1800 • Philadelphia, Pennsylvania, 19103-2899
http://www.oralmaxsurgeryatlas.theclinics.com

ATLAS OF THE ORAL AND MAXILLOFACIAL SURGERY CLINICS OF NORTH AMERICA Volume 32, Number 1
March 2024 ISSN 1061-3315 ISBN-13: 978-0-443-13089-2

Editor: John Vassallo; j.vassallo@elsevier.com
Developmental Editor: Anita Chamoli

© **2024 Elsevier Inc. All rights are reserved, including those for text and data mining, AI training, and similar technologies.**

This periodical and the individual contributions contained in it are protected under copyright by Elsevier, and the following terms and conditions apply to their use:

Photocopying
Single photocopies of single articles may be made for personal use as allowed by national copyright laws. Permission of the Publisher and payment of a fee is required for all other photocopying, including multiple or systematic copying, copying for advertising or promotional purposes, resale, and all forms of document delivery. Special rates are available for educational institutions that wish to make photocopies for non-profit educational classroom use. For information on how to seek permission visit www.elsevier.com/permissions or call: (+44) 1865 843830 (UK)/(+1) 215 239 3804 (USA).

Derivative Works
Subscribers may reproduce tables of contents or prepare lists of articles including abstracts for internal circulation within their institutions. Permission of the Publisher is required for resale or distribution outside the institution. Permission of the Publisher is required for all other derivative works, including compilations and translations (please consult www.elsevier.com/permissions).

Electronic Storage or Usage
Permission of the Publisher is required to store or use electronically any material contained in this periodical, including any article or part of an article (please consult www.elsevier.com/permissions). Except as outlined above, no part of this publication may be reproduced, stored in a retrieval system or transmitted in any form or by any means, electronic, mechanical, photocopying, recording or otherwise, without prior written permission of the Publisher.

Notice
No responsibility is assumed by the Publisher for any injury and/or damage to persons or property as a matter of products liability, negligence or otherwise, or from any use or operation of any methods, products, instructions or ideas contained in the material herein. Because of rapid advances in the medical sciences, in particular, independent verification of diagnoses and drug dosages should be made. Although all advertising material is expected to conform to ethical (medical) standards, inclusion in this publication does not constitute a guarantee or endorsement of the quality or value of such product or of the claims made of it by its manufacturer.

Reprints. For copies of 100 or more of articles in this publication, please contact the Commercial Reprints Department, Elsevier Inc., 360 Park Avenue South, New York, NY 10010-1710. Tel.: 212-633-3874; Fax: 212-633-3820; E-mail: reprints@elsevier.com.

Atlas of the Oral and Maxillofacial Surgery Clinics of North America (ISSN 1061-3315) is published biannually by Elsevier, 360 Park Avenue South, New York, NY 10010-1710. Months of issue are March and September. Periodicals postage paid at New York, NY and additional mailing offices. Subscription prices are $489.00 for international individual, $416.00 for US individual, $429.00 for Canadian individual; $220.00 for international student, $100.00 for US student and Canadian student. For institutional access pricing please contact Customer Service via the contact information below. Foreign air speed delivery is included in all *Clinics* subscription prices. All prices are subject to change without notice. POSTMASTER: Send address changes to *Atlas of the Oral and Maxillofacial Surgery Clinics of North America*, Health Sciences Division, Subscription Customer Service, 3251 Riverport Lane, Maryland Heights, MO 63043. Tel: 1-800-654-2452 (U.S. and Canada); 314-447-8871 (outside U.S. and Canada). Fax: 314-417-8029. E-mail: journalscustomerservice-usa@elsevier.com (for print support); journalsonline support-usa@elsevier.com (for online support).

Atlas of the Oral and Maxillofacial Surgery Clinics of North America is covered in *MEDLINE/PubMed (Index Medicus)*.

Printed in the United States of America.

Contributors

CONSULTING EDITOR

RUI P. FERNANDES, MD, DMD, FACS, FRCS(Ed)
Clinical Professor and Chief, Division of Head and Neck Surgery, Program Director, Head and Neck Oncologic Surgery and Microvascular Reconstruction Fellowship, Departments of Oral and Maxillofacial Surgery, Neurosurgery, and Orthopaedic Surgery and Rehabilitation, University of Florida Health Science Center, University of Florida College of Medicine–Jacksonville, Jacksonville, Florida

EDITORS

EVAN BUSBY, DMD
Assistant Professor, Department of Oral and Maxillofacial Surgery, University of Florida College of Medicine, University of Florida Health Oral and Maxillofacial Surgery, Jacksonville, Florida

TIRBOD FATTAHI, MD, DDS, FACS
Professor and Chair, Department of Oral and Maxillofacial Surgery, University of Florida College of Medicine, University of Florida Health Oral and Maxillofacial Surgery, Jacksonville, Florida

AUTHORS

PHILLIP HOOPER BARBEE, MD, DDS, MS
Surgeon, Facial Plastic and Reconstructive Surgery, Clevens Face and Body Specialists, Melbourne, Florida

EVAN BUSBY, DMD
Assistant Professor, Department of Oral and Maxillofacial Surgery, University of Florida College of Medicine, University of Florida Health Oral and Maxillofacial Surgery, Jacksonville, Florida

CANG CARSON HUYNH, MD, DMD, FACS, FAACS
Private Practice, Radiance Surgery & Aesthetic Medicine, Atlanta, Georgia

ROSS A. CLEVENS, MD, FACS
Fellowship Director, Facial Plastic and Reconstructive Surgery, Clevens Face and Body Specialists, Melbourne, Florida

TIRBOD FATTAHI, MD, DDS, FACS
Professor and Chair, Department of Oral and Maxillofacial Surgery, University of Florida College of Medicine, University of Florida Health Oral and Maxillofacial Surgery, Jacksonville, Florida

ELDA FISHER, DMD, MD, FACS
Associate Professor of Surgery, Division of Plastic, Maxillofacial, and Oral Surgery, Duke University; Adjunct Associate Professor, ASOD–Division of Craniofacial and Surgical Care, The University of North Carolina at Chapel Hill, Chapel Hill, North Carolina

CHRISTOPHER HAMAMDJIAN, DO
Private Practice, Radiance Surgery & Aesthetic Medicine, Atlanta, Georgia

BANG QUACH, MD, DMD
Fellow, Facial Plastic and Reconstructive Surgery, Clevens Face and Body Specialists, Melbourne, Florida

FAISAL A. QUERESHY, MD, DDS
Program Director and Professor, Department of Oral and Maxillofacial Surgery, Case Western Reserve University, Cleveland, Ohio

MAJID REZAEI, DDS MSc
Resident, Department of Oral and Maxillofacial Surgery, College of Medicine, University of Florida Health, Jacksonville, Florida

Contributors

GEORGE F. SCHIEDER IV, DMD
Resident, Department of Oral and Maxillofacial Surgery, Case Western Reserve University, Cleveland, Ohio

MAYA D. SINHA, BS
Emory University School of Medicine, Atlanta, Georgia

PRADEEP K. SINHA, MD, PhD, FACS
Private Practice, Atlanta, Georgia

Contents

Preface   ix

Evan Busby and Tirbod Fattahi

Historical and Biological Properties of Injectables   1

Evan Busby and Tirbod Fattahi

- Introduction   1
- Neurotoxins   1
  - Biology of neurotoxins   1
- Dermal fillers   3
  - Biology of dermal fillers   3
  - Reversal   4
- Summary   5
- Disclosure   5

Applications for Neurotoxins in the Face and Neck   7

Elda Fisher

- Introduction and preoperative planning   7
- Preparation for injection   7
- Supplies   8
- Surgical preparation   8
- Injection technique   9
- Forehead   9
- Glabella   9
- Crow's feet (orbicularis oculi)   10
- Bunny lines   10
- Gummy smile   10
- Lip flip   11
- Lower face contouring/masseter contouring   11
- Marionette lines/depressor anguli oris   11
- Platysmal banding   12
- Complications   12
- Immediate postoperative care   14
- Summary   14
- Clinics care points   14
- Disclosure   14

Injectable Fillers for Lower Face Rejuvenation   15

Majid Rezaei, Evan Busby, and Tirbod Fattahi

- Introduction   15
- Regional anatomy   15
- Injectable fillers   15
- Clinical evaluation   16
- Technique   16
- Mandibular angle   18

Contents

Chin	18
Jowling and prejowl sulcus	20
Complications	21
Clinics care points	21
Disclosure	21

Perioral Filler Augmentation   23
Faisal A. Quereshy and George F. Schieder IV

Introduction	23
Surgical technique	23
Preoperative Planning	23
Prep and Patient Positioning	23
Lip Filler	24
Perioral Vertical Rhytid Filler	25
Nasolabial Fold Filler	27
Marionette Line Filler	29
Mentolabial Filler	29
Postoperative care	29
Potential complications	29
Clinics care points	33
Disclosure	33

Liquid Facelift   35
Maya D. Sinha and Pradeep K. Sinha

Introduction	35
Neurotoxins	35
Dermal Fillers	36
Cautions	40
Summary	40
Clinics care points	40
Disclosure	41

Nonsurgical Rhinoplasty with Hyaluronic Acid   43
Cang Carson Huynh and Christopher Hamamdjian

Introduction: Nature of the Problem	43
Technique	43
Surgical technique	46
Preoperative Planning	46
Prep and Patient Positioning	46
Pearls and Pitfalls	46
Immediate postoperative care	46
Rehabilitation and Recovery	46
Clinical results	46
Summary	46
Clinics care points	47

Periorbital Rejuvenation   49

Phillip Hooper Barbee

Introduction: nature of the problem   49
Upper eyelid rejuvenation   49
Lower eyelid rejuvenation   49
Surgical technique   49
    Preoperative planning   49
    Surgical approach   50
Rehabilitation and recovery   54
Summary   54
Disclosure   54

Complications of Injectables   57

Bang Quach and Ross A. Clevens

Introduction   57
    Complications of neuromodulators   57
    Complications of dermal fillers   59
Summary   63
Disclosure   63

ATLAS OF THE ORAL AND MAXILLOFACIAL SURGERY CLINICS OF NORTH AMERICA

FORTHCOMING ISSUES

September 2024

Maxillary and Midface Reconstruction, Part 1
James C. Melville, Rui P. Fernandes, and Michael R. Markiewicz, *Editors*

March 2025

Maxillary and Midface Reconstruction, Part 2
James C. Melville, Rui P. Fernandes, and Michael R. Markiewicz, *Editors*

PREVIOUS ISSUES

September 2023

Reconstruction of the Mandible
Michael R. Markiewicz, James C. Melville, and Rui P. Fernandes, *Editors*

March 2023

Facial Reanimation
Teresa González Otero, *Editor*

September 2022

Surgical Management of the Temporomandibular Joint
Florencio Monje, *Editor*

SERIES OF RELATED INTEREST

Oral and Maxillofacial Surgery Clinics
http://www.oralmaxsurgery.theclinics.com/

Dental Clinics
http://www.dental.theclinics.com

THE CLINICS ARE NOW AVAILABLE ONLINE!

Access your subscription at:
www.theclinics.com

Preface

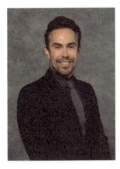
Evan Busby, DMD

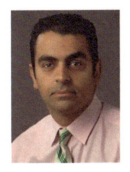
Tirbod Fattahi, MD, DDS, FACS

Editors

We are delighted to bring to you the latest issue of the *Atlas of Oral & Maxillofacial Surgery Clinics of North America*. In this issue, devoted entirely to dermal fillers and cosmetic neurotoxins, a comprehensive overview and clinical applications of these products are presented. Considering the worldwide utilization and demand of dermal fillers and cosmetic neurotoxins, along with the evolving utilization of noninvasive facial rejuvenative procedures, this *Atlas of Oral & Maxillofacial Surgery Clinics of North America* could not get published soon enough!

Each article includes the author's specific preference for application of these noninvasive procedures for facial rejuvenation. In addition to understanding the history and biomechanical properties of fillers and neurotoxins, attention is also directed toward application of these products for specific parts of the face; "liquid" face lifting and "liquid" rhinoplasty are just two examples of this.

Other articles are skillfully designed to aid the reader in understanding the "how-to" techniques and to familiarize the audience with pearls and potential pitfalls. There is also an entire article on the management of complications of dermal fillers and neurotoxins.

We are both so grateful for the support and invitation from the editorial board of the *Atlas of Oral & Maxillofacial Surgery Clinics of North America* (Dr Rui Fernandes, Mr John Vassallo, and administrative staff). We are also indebted to our colleagues and friends who have contributed to the creation of this issue of the *Atlas of Oral & Maxillofacial Surgery Clinics of North America*.

Sincerely,

Evan Busby, DMD
University of Florida College of Medicine
Department of Oral & Maxillofacial Surgery
UF Health Oral and Maxillofacial Surgery
3rd Floor, Faculty Clinic
653 West 8th Street
Jacksonville, FL 32209, USA

Tirbod Fattahi, MD, DDS, FACS
University of Florida College of Medicine
Department of Oral & Maxillofacial Surgery
UF Health Oral and Maxillofacial Surgery
3rd Floor, Faculty Clinic
653 West 8th Street
Jacksonville, FL 32209, USA

E-mail addresses:
evan.busby@jax.ufl.edu (E. Busby)
tirbod.fattahi@jax.ufl.edu (T. Fattahi)

Historical and Biological Properties of Injectables

Evan Busby, DMD[a], Tirbod Fattahi, DDS, MD, FACS[b,*]

KEYWORDS

- Neurotoxins • Dermal fillers • Injectable physiology

KEY POINTS

- Since their introduction in the United States in the early 2000s, cosmetic neurotoxins and dermal fillers have become the most popular nonsurgical modalities in facial cosmetic surgery.
- The purpose of this article is to familiarize the reader with a brief history as well as the biochemical and physiologic properties of the most commonly used cosmetic neurotoxins and dermal fillers.
- Cosmetic neurotoxins and dermal fillers are extremely popular in the facial cosmetic surgery arena.

Introduction

Since their introduction in the United States in the early 2000s, cosmetic neurotoxins and dermal fillers have become the most popular nonsurgical modalities in facial cosmetic surgery. Cosmetic surgery (total body including the face) is a 20-billion-dollar industry in our country, of which roughly 25% is attributed to neurotoxins (onabotulinumtoxinA [Botox Cosmetic], abobotulinumtoxinA [Dysport], incobotulinumtoxinA [Xeomin]) and various types of semi-permanent and permanent dermal fillers (ie, hyaluronic acid gel [Juvederm], non-animal stabilized hyaluronic acid (NASHA) [Restylane], injectable poly-L-lactic acid [Sculptra], silicone, and so forth) (Fig. 1).

The purpose of this article is to familiarize the reader with a brief history as well as the biochemical and physiologic properties of the most commonly used cosmetic neurotoxins and dermal fillers.

Neurotoxins

Since their inception in Belgium after an outbreak of food (sausage) poisoning in the late 1800s (*botulus* is Latin for sausage), botulinum neurotoxins (BoNTs) have been around and studied for various purposes. BoNTs come from gram-positive anaerobic bacteria *Clostridium botulinum* and are actually exotoxins and not a true infection. It has been reported that the US military actually experimented with various BoNTs as a biological weapon around World War II. There are multiple types of BoNTs; however, type A is the most potent and the one used primarily for medical purposes. Around the late 1960s and 1970s, the medical benefits of botulinum were established in the management of strabismus and blepharospasm. Oculinum Inc. became the first American company to manufacture botulinum toxin A (BTA) for the treatment of blepharospasm. In 1989, Allergan purchased Oculinum and began to produce BTA for functional purposes (strabismus correction and blepharospasm). In the early 1990s, 2 Canadian physicians, Dr Jean and Dr Alastair Carruthers, discovered the cosmetic benefits of BTA which eventually led to the creation of what we today refer to as "Botox Cosmetic." The Food and Drug Administration (FDA) finally approved onabotulinumtoxinA (Botox) in the United States for glabellar wrinkles in 2002.

Biology of neurotoxins

All type A neurotoxins (currently onabotulinumtoxinA [Botox Cosmetic], abobotulinumtoxinA [Dysport], Dysport], incobotulinumtoxinA [Xeomin]) work by blocking the release of acetylcholine from the presynaptic receptors of muscle fibers. Specifically, the SNARE (SNAp [soluble N-ethylmaleimide-sensitive factor-attachment protein] REceptor) protein is cleaved by onabotulinumtoxinA (Botox), thereby blocking muscle contraction (Fig. 2). OnabotulinumtoxinA (Botox) only works on new acetylcholine receptors with no effect on circulating acetylcholine receptors, hence the delay of onset of 3 to 5 days. Typical duration of most neurotoxins is about 3 months; this occurs after the body begins to produce new acetylcholine receptors which overpower the residual effects of onabotulinumtoxinA (Botox).

All neurotoxins come in a powdered form and require reconstitution with preservative-free saline (Fig. 3). Some have recommended the use of lidocaine for reconstitution to diminish pain on injection. While sterile water has been used by some, it should never be used due to a lack of physiologic pH balance and intense pain upon injection. Although multiple constitution ratios are used, both authors advocate the most basic and consistent mixture ratio (Fig. 4).

---

[a] Department of Oral & Maxillofacial Surgery, University of Florida College of Medicine, 1710 Challen Avenue, Jacksonville, FL 32205, USA
[b] Department of Oral & Maxillofacial Surgery, University of Florida College of Medicine, Jacksonville
* Corresponding author. University of Florida, 653-1 West 8th Street, Jacksonville, FL 32209.
E-mail address: tirbod.fattahi@jax.ufl.edu

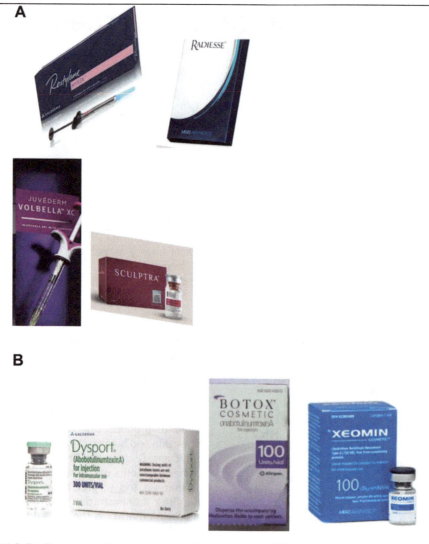

Fig. 1 (*A* & *B*). Examples of the most commonly used dermal fillers and neurotoxins. (From: AbbVie.)

Dermal fillers

Injectable dermal fillers date back to the late 1970s in the United States. The original injectable fillers were comprised of bovine collagen and while quite popular, caused a whole host of allergic reactions which eventually led to the downfall of animal-based injectables. In the 1980s and 1990s, fat injection and transfer almost replaced the need for bovine-based injectables. With the aid of new instrumentation, the advent of tumescent anesthesia, and newer surgical techniques such as Coleman's fat transfer method, fat injection and fat transfer became quite popular. However, as popular as fat injection was and still is today, there was a clear need for another form of injectable product that was consistent, safe, nonallergenic and did not require the need for an additional harvesting procedure. This void led to the creation of the first generation of NASHA. Hyaluronic acid (HA) is a hydrophilic protein found abundantly in skin and within joint spaces throughout the body. Due to the molecular weight of the protein particles and its unique hydrophilic properties, HA maintains moisture and displays a lubricating effect, hence its popular utilization in sports medicine and intracapsular joint injections (Fig. 5). NASHA (Restylane) became the first HA filler in the United States in 2003 and to this day, stills holds tremendous popularity amongst clinicians.

Dermal fillers are essentially divided into 2 categories:

- HA fillers (hyaluronic acid gel [Juvederm], NASHA [Restylane], NASHA [Perlane], and so forth)
- Non-HA fillers (calcium hydroxylapatite [Radiesse], injectable poly-L-lactic acid [Sculptra], silicone, and so forth)

Dermal fillers are also categorized based on the "permanency" of the product. Essentially, all HA fillers are considered "non-permanent" or "semi-permanent" whereas all non-HA fillers are considered "permanent" although there is quite a bit of variability in the duration and longevity of the "permanent" fillers. Of significant clinical importance is the fact that only HA fillers can be reversed with an "antidote"; permanent fillers do not have a reversal agent. This principle should be considered when a novice injector is contemplating using dermal fillers. Since HA fillers are considered the most popular and most widely used fillers in the cosmetic arena, the biological properties of HA will be further discussed in this *Atlas* article.

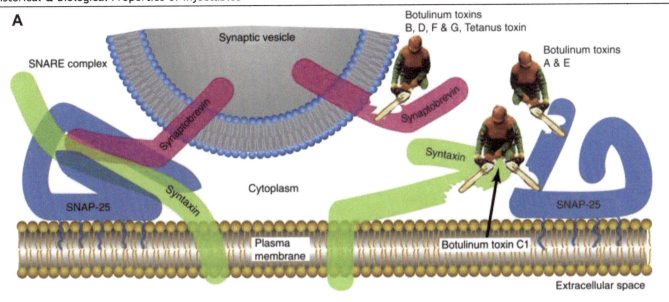
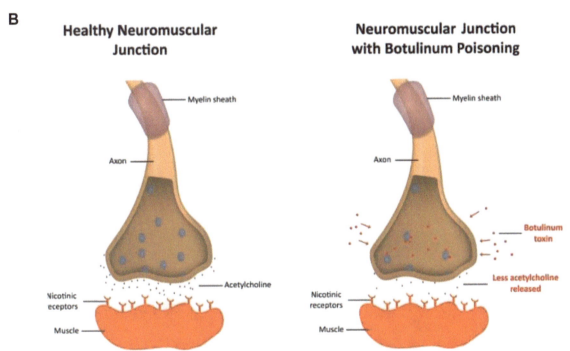

Fig. 2 (*A* and *B*). Mechanism of action of botulinum toxin. Note interaction of SNARE protein within the synaptic membrane prior to cleavage by the exotoxin (*A*) and blockage of release of acetylcholine by botulinum toxin (*B*). SNARE, SNAp (soluble N-ethylmaleimide-sensitive factor-attachment protein) REceptor. (Fig. 2(*A*) *From*: Thomas L. Schwarz. Release of Neurotransmitters, in Fundamental Neuroscience (Fourth Edition), 2013, Fig. 7.5. Fig. 2(*B*) *From*: Botulinum Toxin, Sarah Knapp Reviewed by BD Editors. Last Updated: October 4, 2020. https://biologydictionary.net/botulinum-toxin/.)

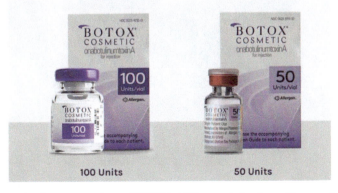

Fig. 3 (Botox Cosmetic) in its 2 concentrations. (BOTOX®. With permission from Allergan, Inc., an AbbVie company.)

Added Normal Saline	50U Vial Botox Concentration	100U Vial Botox Concentration
1.0 cc	5U/0.1 cc	-
2.0 cc	-	5U/0.1 cc

Fig. 4 The preferred method of mixing onabotulinumtoxinA (Botox) by the authors.

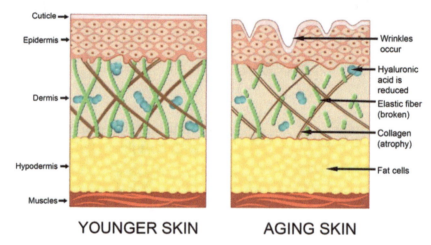

Fig. 5 Hydrophilic properties of HA molecules within skin; note the "smoothing" and lubricating effect of HA particles within the skin. (*From*: https://www.therefineryskinclinic.com/hydrate-with-hyaluronic-acid/.)

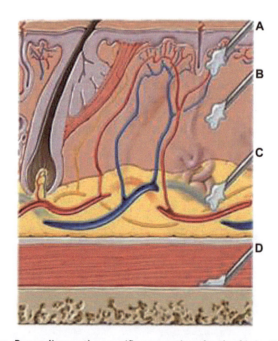

Fig. 6 Various sites of injection of fillers. Depending on the specific properties, depth of injection needs to be modified. (Joe Niamtu, 10 - Injectable Fillers: Lip Augmentation, Lip Reduction, and Lip Lift, in Joe Niamtu, Cosmetic Facial Surgery (Second Edition), Elsevier, 2018.)

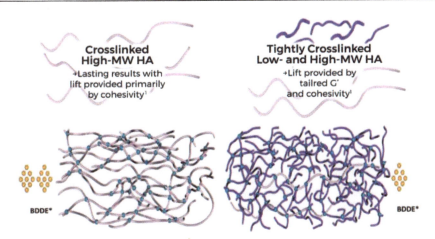

Fig. 7 Cross-linking of hyaluronic acid (HA) particles in order to create a more viscous hydrogel. (With permission from Clinic RX. Figure retrieved *from*: https://www.clinicrx.com.my/the-caseforjuvederm/.)

Biology of dermal fillers

Regardless of the degree of permanency or presence of HA particles, dermal fillers add volume to the injected site. They "fill" a groove or trough or wrinkle and enhance the volume of a particular area. The term "dermal fillers" is a bit of a misnomer since not all fillers are injected into the dermis. The biological properties of the specific filler determine its ideal location (dermis vs supraperiosteal) (Fig. 6).

HA fillers are manufactured by fermentation of specific bacterial species in order to create an HA molecule. Once the HA molecule has been created, it is stabilized by a process called cross-linking to other HA molecules; this creates a hydrogel product which when injected into the body, prevents the immediate absorption of the HA particle (Fig. 7).

HA fillers are categorized based on the following:

- Particle size and flow (rheology)
- Concentration of HA molecules
- Degree of cross-linking
- Degree of hydrophilic properties

Particle size impacts the rheology of dermal fillers. Fillers with smaller particle sizes also tend to be less viscous and easier to inject. For example, Juvederm Volbella XC (hyaluronic acid gel) has a very small particle size (around 250 nm), is quite soft, and easy to inject and therefore more appropriate for thinner skin areas such as the lips and lower lids. On the other hand, larger particle-size fillers (Juvederm Voluma XC [hyaluronic acid gel],-for example) have significantly larger particle sizes (up to 800 nm) and are far more viscous and therefore should not be used in thinner areas of the face. These large-sized and viscous fillers are more appropriate for deeper injections (preperiosteal). Furthermore, the higher the concentration of HA molecules per gram of filler, the more hydrophilic the filler becomes. Fillers with more hydrophilic properties (more concentrated) also tend to have more cross-linking of the HA particles which in turn increases the longevity of the product. Increased cross-linking also increases the viscosity of the filler, hence affecting its rheology.

Regardless of the degree of cross-linking, at some point the body begins to breakdown the HA particles and the surrounding hydrogel, hence eliminating the volumetric benefits of fillers. This process may be as short as a few months for less viscous and small particle-size fillers, all the way to a year for large particle-size fillers that are also more cross-linked.

Reversal

Perhaps one of the greatest benefits of HA fillers is the availability of an antidote. Synthetic reversal enzyme for HA particles, hyaluronidase (Vitrase or Hylenex) is an injectable solution which begins to almost immediately break down HA molecules. This is of significant clinical value for both early and late potential complications associated with HA fillers.

Summary

Cosmetic neurotoxins and dermal fillers are extremely popular in the facial cosmetic surgery arena. Understanding the biological mechanism of these products can enhance the clinician's comfort and willingness to incorporate these products into their everyday cosmetic practice.

Disclosure

None.

Further Reading

Herrmann JL, Hoffmann RK, Ward CE, et al. Biochemistry, physiology, and tissue interactions of contemporary biodegradable injectable dermal fillers. Dermatol Surg 2018;44(Suppl 1):S19–31.

Keen MA. Hyaluronic acid in dermatology. Skinmed 2017;15(6):441–8.

Bass LS. Injectable filler techniques for facial rejuvenation, volumization, and augmentation. Facial Plast Surg Clin North Am 2015; 23(4):479–88.

Funt D, Pavicic T. Dermal fillers in aesthetics: an overview of adverse events and treatment approaches. Plast Surg Nurs 2015;35(1):13–32.

Pierre S, Liew S, Bernardin A. Basics of dermal filler rheology. Dermatol Surg 2015;41(Suppl 1):S120–6.

Tighe AP, Schiavo G. Botulinum neurotoxins: mechanism of action. Toxicon 2013;67:87–93.

Swift A, Green JB, Hernandez CA, et al. Tips and tricks for facial toxin injections with Illustrated anatomy. Plast Reconstr Surg 2022; 149(2):303e–12e.

Kroumpouzos G, Kassir M, Gupta M, et al. Complications of Botulinum toxin A: an update review. J Cosmet Dermatol 2021;20(6):1585–90. Epub 2021 Apr 30. PMID: 33864431.

Applications for Neurotoxins in the Face and Neck

Elda Fisher, DMD, MD [a,b,*]

KEYWORDS

- Botox • Dysport • Xeomin • Jeuveau • Daxxify • Neurotoxin • Esthetic medicine • Botox brow lift

KEY POINTS

- There are several commercially available neurotoxins for esthetic enhancement of the face and neck.
- Although Food and Drug Administration-approved neurotoxins are commercially available for injections in several regions of the upper face, there are esthetic applications for their use in the mid-face, lower-face, and neck.
- The use of neurotoxins for esthetic enhancement yields subtle and temporary effects.
- When planning for neurotoxin injections, it is critical to capture preinjection clinical photos of the patient for reference.
- Complications with the use of neurotoxins are minimal and typically temporary.

Introduction and preoperative planning

Patient selection is crucial when considering neurotoxin treatment of esthetic improvement. Neurotoxins effectively target dynamic wrinkles, which are caused by the normal functioning of facial muscles. However, it is important to note that deep lines, wrinkles, and crevasses in the face are not effectively treated with neurotoxins. Some patients may visit the office seeking nonsurgical rejuvenation and may ask for "Botox" without realizing that it differs from fillers. Similarly, some patients may desire nonsurgical correction of facial wrinkles despite having deep and long-standing wrinkles due to advanced aging and volume loss.

In general, neurotoxins provide subtle yet noticeable improvements in mimetic lines, commonly observed in patients aged younger than 50 years. However, for patients aged older than 50 years, relying solely on neurotoxins is unlikely to sufficiently address their primary concerns.

Several neurotoxin products are available, each with unique properties and characteristics. The most commonly used neurotoxins in esthetic medicine include botulinum toxin type A formulations such as Botox, Dysport, Xeomin, and Jeuveau. Although all these products share the common mechanism of temporarily inhibiting muscle contractions, there are subtle differences among them.

Botox, the pioneering and widely recognized neurotoxin, has a well-established track record in the field. Dysport is another botulinum toxin type A formulation that has been in use for almost 20 years and has gained popularity due to its slightly more rapid onset of action. Xeomin, a more recent addition, is a botulinum toxin that undergoes a unique purification process, making it free from complexing proteins. Jeuveau is one the newest botulinum toxins and is purported to last longer than the other available options. Xeomin and Jeuveau do not require refrigeration before reconstitution, which may make these products more attractive to a traveling practitioner or one with limited medical refrigerator space.

Although these neurotoxin formulations have distinct characteristics, it is important to note that they all share the overall objective of reducing dynamic facial wrinkles and achieving facial rejuvenation. The selection of a specific neurotoxin product depends on factors such as practitioner preference, clinical experience, and patient expectations.

Differences in dosing, reconstitution, and diffusion patterns also exist among these neurotoxin products. The units used for dosing may vary, making it crucial for health-care professionals to understand the conversion ratios when switching between products. Table 1 illustrates the various products, their reconstitution, storage, and longevity based on the manufacturer's guidelines, and this authors reconstitution and storage, which may differ from package inserts and manufactures specifications.

Preparation for injection

In all cases, the patient should be aware of the effect, both intended and unintended, of the neurotoxin. A thorough discussion of likely cosmetic outcomes, timing, and duration of effect, along with risks and benefits should occur with each patient before injection and be included on the consent forms. Specifically, the patient should be warned about allergic reactions, dissatisfaction with esthetic result, lid ptosis, brow drooping, and general effect on nearby muscle groups. Contraindications to the use of neurotoxins are musculoskeletal diseases such as Lambert-Eaton Disease, myasthenia gravis, and amyotrophic lateral sclerosis (ALS). The most common relative contraindications to treatment are age less than 18 years, pregnancy, and previous allergic reaction to another neurotoxin.

---

[a] Division of Plastic, Maxillofacial, and Oral Surgery, Duke University
[b] ASOD — Division of Craniofacial and Surgical Care, University of North Carolina at Chapel Hill, 149 Brauer Hall, CB 7450, Chapel Hill, NC 27599, USA
* Corresponding author. Division of Plastic, Maxillofacial and Ora Surgery, Duke University Medical Center, Box 2955, Durham, NC 27710.
E-mail address: Elda.fisher@Duke.edu

Table 1 Various products, their reconstitution, storage, and longevity based on the manufacturer's guidelines

Product	Diluent	Recommended dilution	Alternative dilution	Recommended dose to treat glabellar lines
Botox	Preservative free 0.9% sodium chloride	100 U/2.5 mL	100 U/1 mL	20 U
Dysport	Preservative free 0.9% sodium chloride	300 U/2.5 mL	300 U/1 mL	60 U
Jeuveau	Preservative free 0.9% sodium chloride	100 U/2.5 mL	100 U/1 mL	20 U
Xeomin	Preservative free 0.9% sodium chloride	Varies	100 U/1 mL	20 U
Daxxify	Preservative free 0.9% sodium chloride	100 U/1.2 mL	100 U/1 mL	40 U

Photograph documentation is also a priority for these patients. Although this is cumbersome and time consuming, many patients will point out postprocedure "changes" that were actually present before injections. It is important to keep these records so that both you and the patient can evaluate your outcomes objectively (Fig. 1).

Supplies

Manufacturers of neurotoxins for esthetic use generally recommend the use of 27-gauge needles for injection after reconstitution. This author routinely uses 31gauge needles because these are less painful to the patient on injection (Fig. 2). The smaller bore needles, however, make it more difficult to draw up the reconstituted medication into the syringe. Needles should be used only for up 3 sites because smaller bore needles tend to dull and become more painful with each injection. Similarly, when drawing up the medication from the vial, the rubber stopper should be entered without bending the needle and should only be used to pierce the rubber stopper once, as this also dulls the needle. Before use, the rubber stopper should be cleaned with an alcohol wipe.

Surgical preparation

After obtaining consent and photograph documentation, it is time to prepare the patient. The patient should be in a reclined position for injections. Clean the intended area with

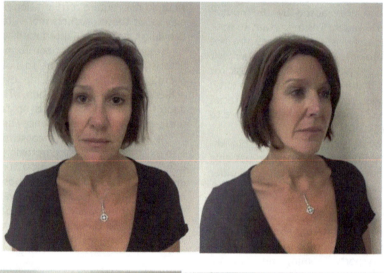
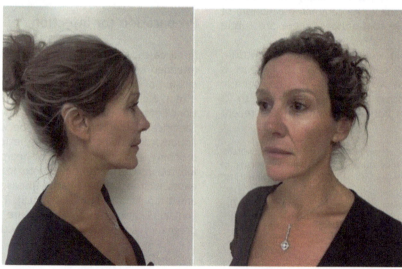

Fig. 1 Photographs for documentation.

Applications for Neurotoxins in the Face and Neck

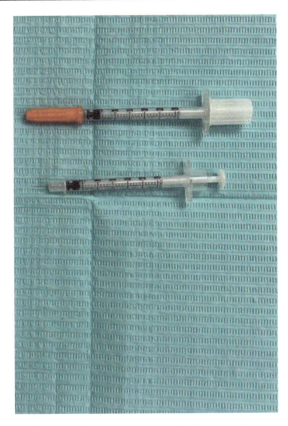

Figs. 2 The 31-gauge needles for injection.

alcohol wipes and check to make sure the wipe is clean before proceeding (remove all dirt and makeup). A make-up pencil can be used to mark the sites for injection but the injections should not travel through the marks but rather adjacent to them to avoid deposition of the makeup pencil marking into the dermis (Fig. 3A–C).

Injection technique

In all areas, the injection technique follows the same principles with one exception, in some areas, it is easier to pinch the skin for injection, and in some areas, it is better to stretch the skin and inject into the stretched area (Fig. 4A–B). Some texts recommend inserting the needle to the bone, and then backing out a small amount to inject supraperiosteally. This recommendation is based on the knowledge that all but 4 of the muscles of facial expression are innervated from their deep surface. The technique of contacting the periosteum is painful for patients and can be avoided by injection just deep to the dermis because there is no benefit to efficacy or longevity of the product with deeper injection.

Forehead

Horizontal forehead rhytids are a common chief complaint of patients seeking cosmetic improvement with neurotoxins. It is important to remember that the horizontal forehead rhytids are the result of contraction of the frontalis muscle, which is the only elevator of the brows. It is important to treat the areas exerting downward force on the brows (glabella, crow's feet) in all patients seeking correction of horizontal forehead rhytids. If the forehead is treated without concomitant treatment of the depressor muscles of the forehead, the patient will experience obvious brow depression and may also develop a forehead bulge in the brow region. Patients with deep forehead rhytids often depend on frontalis muscle activity to see clearly in superior gaze. As such although it is tempting to treat patients with deep forehead rhytids with higher doses of neurotoxin, this is ill-advised because the patient will likely notice significant brow ptosis and may even find difficulty elevating their brows, which is distressing. This author recommends treatment of the forehead with the lowest dose possible to obtain the desired esthetic outcome with the longest duration. The recommended dosing varies from different manufacturers.

Patients seeking feminine brow contours generally prefer an arched brow, whereas a more masculine appearance is typically associated with more horizontal positioning of the brows. To maintain the arch of the brow, it is again important to remember that the frontalis is the only elevator of the brow, and there is benefit in delivering lower doses of neurotoxin in the frontalis lateral to the planned brow apex in comparison to the frontalis at the medial brow to limit depression of the apex and tail of the brow (see Fig. 3B and C).

Delivery to the frontalis should span the forehead, and in patients with long foreheads, it may be necessary to perform 3 rows of injections instead of 2 as this author typically recommends.

Glabella

The glabella region of the forehead has 2 muscles groups both contributing to depression of the brows. The corrugator muscles are oriented nearly horizontally in the medial half of each brow, with the inferior aspect more medial and the superior aspect of the muscle more lateral.

The procerus muscle is a midline muscle contracting toward the nasal radix and, therefore, contributing to depression of the medial brows (Fig. 5A–B).

This muscle group at the glabella is treated as one region. Patients seeking improvement in this area may complain of vertical glabellar rhytids ("11s" or "angry lines") or may complain of a horizontal rhytid just superior to the nasal radix.

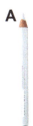 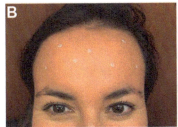 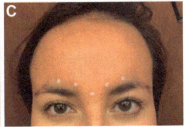

Fig. 3 (A) Makeup pencil. (B, C) Brow contours.

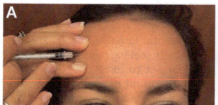 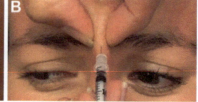

Fig. 4 Injection technique. (*A*) Skin stretch. (*B*) Skin pinch.

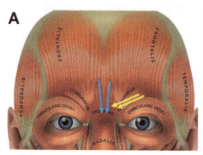 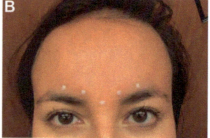

Figs. 5 (*A*, *B*) Corrugator muscles and procerus muscles.

Because the corrugator muscles run in a horizontally directed manner (see Fig. 5), this author typically injects along the length of the medial muscle. A smaller and more superficial injection is then performed at lateral aspect of the corrugator. It is wise to inject a lower dose and more superficially at the lateral corrugator because this injection has the highest risk of dispersion deep and inferior to affect the levator muscle of the eyelid, producing a complication of true lid ptosis.

The procerus can be injected at one point or at 2 locations vertical to each other approximately 1 cm apart.

Crow's feet (orbicularis oculi)

The lateral canthal rhytids commonly described as "crow's feet" are the mimetic rhytids caused by contraction of the vertical portion of the lateral aspect of the orbicularis oculi muscles. When the orbicularis contracts, the brow and specifically the tail of the brow is depressed. Treatment of the lateral canthal lines with neurotoxin will produce some degree of brow elevation. This is generally a desired effect, and commonly referred to colloquially as a "Botox" brow lift, because paralysis of these vertical fibers will leave the upward movement by the frontalis unopposed. Many patients present with a desire to treat these crow's feet rhytids and have a simultaneous brow lift; however, the practitioner should use caution when treating these muscles. Although enough neurotoxin to remove lines at rest is desireable, too much will remove all vertical component contraction of the small orbicularis muscle, and patients will look alien and abnormal on animation (ie, it is unnatural looking for an adult woman to smile and have no "smile lines" or mimetic lines at this site). When treating this area, the patient should be advised that a natural look is desired, and the goal should not be to fully paralyze this area.

In some patients, "crow's feet" extend inferolaterally. In these cases, typically the contraction of the zygomaticus musculature is contributing to the appearance of these lines. It is important to avoid paralysis of the origin of the zygomaticus major because this is just deep and slightly inferolateral to the orbicularis. Paralysis of the zygomaticus major will result in changes in the patient's smile, and this is undesirable.

This author typically injects one-third of the recommended dose equally divided into 2 to 3 distinct sites at the orbicularis. The injections are very superficial because deep injections here can result in bruising secondary to branches of the sentinel vein. One injection is at the tail of the brow, one directly in to the most horizontal rhytid, and if necessary, one at slightly more inferior horizontal rhytid. Injecting one-third of the manufacturer recommended dose ensures a natural looking smile while still providing the effect of minimizing static crow's feet (Fig. 6A–D).

Bunny lines

"Bunny lines" are the diagonally oriented lines caused by action of the alaeque nasi muscle at the origin at the medial aspect of the maxilla. This muscle, which acts as an elevator of the lip, is contracted when a patient is the action of sniffing. Treatment of these lines can be difficult because the alaeque nasi is a powerful muscle and acts to elevate the upper lip. Adequate paralysis at the origin to remove bunny lines will result in depression of the upper lip and decreased tooth show. Targeting an incisor tooth display at rest of 2 to 3 mm in a female patient is ideal; therefore, patients who present with 2 mm incisor show and want neurotoxin treatment for bunny lines should be warned that adequate treatment of the bunny lines will likely result in decreased incisor show and an overall more aged appearance. I typically recommend reducing these bunny lines with a small amount of neurotoxin (2–3 Botox equivalents per side aimed perpendicular to the skin at the origin of the alaeque nasi and junction of the nasalis) and advise the patient that the goal is to reduce the appearance of the these lines at rest but he/she should not expect complete resolution (Fig. 7B).

Gummy smile

A gummy smile is a common complaint, particularly for those with vertical maxillary excess. For ideal esthetics in a feminine patient, the central incisor should demonstrate 2 to 3 mm incisal show at rest, and at full smile the entire tooth and 1 to

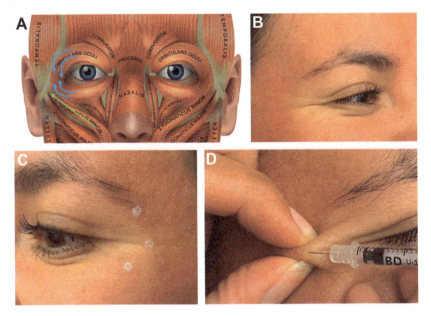

Fig. 6 (*A*) Orbicularis oculi and course of sentinel vein. (*B, C*) Injection pattern at orbicularis. (*D*) Injection of orbicularis.

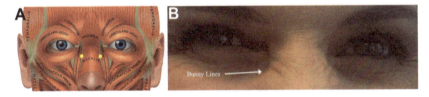

Fig. 7 (*A*) Levator labii alaeque nasi with injection sites. (*B*) Bunny lines.

2 mm gingiva may show. Gingival show beyond 1 to 2 mm is considered excessive and is usually amenable to neurotoxin treatment. The primary elevator of the lip is the levator labii alaeque nasi. Ideal placement of neurotoxin can be palpated approximately 1 cm lateral to the lateral aspect of the nasal ala. This author typically starts with 2 to 3 Botox equivalents per side. On occasion one side elevates higher than the other, and treatment should be customized to more neurotoxin in the hyper functional side (Fig. 8A–C).

Lip flip

Injections into the orbicularis oris have been popularized on social media, and as a result, many patients come to the office requesting a "lip flip." It is important to stress to the patient that neurotoxin treatment of the orbicularis will produce very subtle changes in vermillion and does not reproduce the effects of lip filler or other lip augmentation procedures. The orbicularis oris is a sphincter muscle of the lip, and the lip flip procedure is directed at the horizontal and inferior fibers at the superior vermillion margin. Paralysis of this section of the orbicularis encourages vermillion eversion and results in greater vermillion show. Patients should be aware that the orbicularis is a highly used muscle in all people, and the functional effects of neurotoxin are in almost all cases noticed by patients. As such, they should be warned that it may be difficult to use straws, play certain musical instruments, or whistle. The skin should be stretched before injection, and the needle should enter at the white roll and inserted approximately 2 to 3 mm in a superomedial direction. This author typically starts with 2 Botox equivalents at the cupids bow bilaterally, and 1 Botox equivalent at the lateral injections sites. This dose can be increased up to a total of 10 to 12 total units but patients should be cautioned that injection of more than 6 to 8 units will cause functional changes and hypomobility of the upper lip (Fig. 9A–B).

Lower face contouring/masseter contouring

For patients presenting with hypertrophic masseter muscles, in many cases resulting in square/masculine lower facial third, treatment of the masseter muscles with neurotoxin is an excellent option to produce the desired lower face tapering to restore a feminine facial contour. It is important to advise patients that treatment with neurotoxins is always temporary, and once the neurotoxin has worn off, the masseters will generally return after 1 to 2 months to it hypertrophic state. As a result, it is important to return for repeat injections regularly to maintain the effect. It is also important to explain to the patient that the masseter muscle is a muscle of mastication, and as such masticatory forces will be weakened, and this may be more apparent on one side or another, and may cause minor changes in occlusion that are perceptible during the onset phase of the neurotoxin's effect.

For injection, the masseter is palpated and typically 2 to 3 sites of maximal contraction are identified. Sites should remain inferior to a line drawn from the tragus to lateral commissure of the lip to avoid neurotoxin spread to the risorius and cause changes in the patient's smile. Typical dosing for injection of the masseter are between 25 and 45 Botox equivalent units per side (Fig. 10A–C).

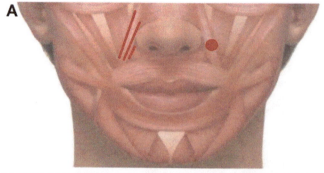
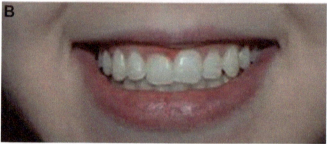
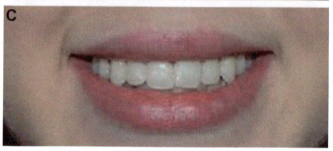

Fig. 8 Treatment of gummy smile. (*A*) Levator Labii with marked injection site (*B/C*) Levator labii before and after injections.

Marionette lines/depressor anguli oris

Obvious marionette lines are typically treated with modalities other than neurotoxin, such as filler placement or facelifting procedures. Minor improvements in down turned lip commissures can be obtained with neurotoxin injections to the depressor anguli oris muscles. The depressor anguli oris is the depressor of the lip commissures, originating at the modiolus and inserting in the mandible just posterior to the insertion of the depressor labii oris. This anatomy is important because inadvertent injection or diffusion of neurotoxin into the labii inferioris will inhibit the natural eversion of the lower lip when eating, particularly food such as sandwiches, where lower lip eversion is necessary to avoid lower lip contacting the lower incisor teeth. To avoid this complication, injections should be placed inferiorly, on the bony insertion, posterior to the depressor labii insertion and approximately 1 cm anterior to the anterior border of the masseter muscle. About 3 to 4 Botox equivalents per side is typical dosing for this area (Fig. 11A–C).

Platysmal banding

As the neck ages, platysmal laxity in some areas contrasted by contraction in others areas leads to platysmal banding and an aged appearance of the neck. Two techniques are useful for treatment of banding, the simplest technique is to pinch the margin of the band with 2 fingers and inject 2 Botox equivalents from the superior aspect of the band continuing inferiorly every 1.5 to 2 cm with additional 2 units until the entire length of the band has been treated. Additional microinjections of 0.25 U along the inferior border of the mandible can also improve the mandibular soft tissue contours. In total, the neck typically has 4 prominent bands, each requiring 8 to 10 units of neurotoxin (Fig. 12A and B).

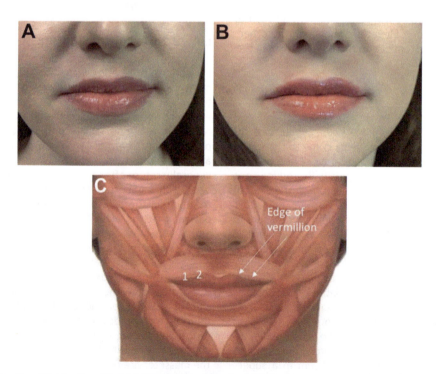

Fig. 9 (*A*) Lip flip. (*B*) Orbicularis oris marked with injection sites. (*C*) Before and after.

Applications for Neurotoxins in the Face and Neck

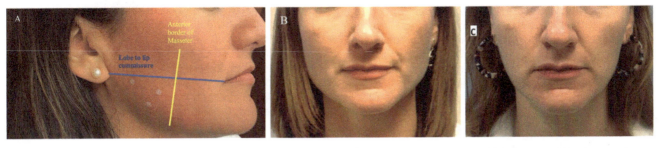

Fig. 10 (A) Masseter Muscle schematic. (B) Sites for injection. (C) Before and after Masseter injections for hypertrophy.

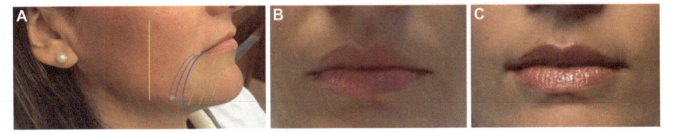

Fig. 11 (A) Depressor anguli oris and depressor labii inferioris. (B) Identification of injection location on skin. (C) Before and after DAO injections. DAO, depressor anguli oris.

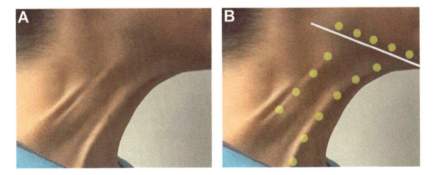

Fig. 12 (A) Platysmal banding. (B) Injection sites for platysmal banding and microbotox along mandibular inferior border.

Complications

Asymmetry: Asymmetries after initial treatment with neurotoxins are common. Even when exact dosing is used symmetrically, overaction or preferred use of one side versus the other can often expose asymmetries. It is important to reassure patients who are new to your practice that asymmetries may be expected at 2 weeks, and a follow-up visit for touchup is important. It is also important to consider that corrections of asymmetries can only be corrected with the addition of more neurotoxin to the opposite side. As an example, patients who are experiencing heavy brows after forehead treatment with neurotoxin (often described as difficulty putting eye makeup on one side) will present to the office with the request to "lift" the affected side. Apart from adding additional neurotoxin to the depressor muscles (corrugators, procerus, and orbicularis), which will typically provide only minimal brow elevation, the option for asymmetry correction is to add more neurotoxin to the appropriately elevated side, which will result in bilateral depression of the brows, a result which is typically unwanted by the patient.

Allergy: Few patients develop allergy to neurotoxins; however, they do occur and are most often caused from the protein complexed to the neurotoxin. Typical presentation is erythema and pruritis in the injected area. Treatment is typically antihistamine, topical steroid cream, or oral steroids depending on the severity of the reaction.

Eyelid ptosis: True lid ptosis should be distinguished from brow lowering and concomitant redundancy of the eyelid skin. In true ptosis, the margin reflex distance is decreased on the affected side secondary to diffusion of neurotoxin in the levator palpebrae muscle. This complication is typically distressing to patients but fortunately self-limited and usually lasting 3 to 4 weeks at most. During that time, patients can be prescribed apraclonidine 0.5% drops to activate Mueller's muscle and increase eyelid opening.

"Spok-like" brows/peakedbrow: This results from inadequate neurotoxin to the superior-lateral forehead. It is corrected by adding 1 to 2 Botox equivalents to the forehead 1.5 to 2 cm directly superior to the over elevated portion of the brow.

Dissatisfaction with esthetic result: This is by far the most common "complication" of neurotoxin treatment. The best and most effective way to prevent this complication is to set patient expectations correctly, reinforcing the idea that neurotoxin treatment is not a facelift, and is not filler. It is designed to make subtle changes in mimetic rhytids, and it does not volumize or remove static rhytids or those caused by damaged skin. Similarly, despite the word "lift" in many treatments, the lifting effect is typically very subtle, and this should be the patient's expectation. Some patients will come in to the office pointing to a particular area posttreatment where they have dissatisfaction. In many cases, this problem was present pretreatment, and so pretreatment photos are absolutely crucial to address these patient concerns.

Immediate postoperative care

Nothing special is necessary for postoperative care. Bruising may be treated with topical arnica gel. Patients can apply makeup as usual, and wash their faces as usual. Some texts recommend that patients do not go to bed or lie on one side of their face as the product may diffuse—this seems intuitively more likely for more dilute concentrations because there is more solution available for diffusion through tissue planes.

Summary

Neurotoxins can be used in the upper, middle, lower face, and neck to achieve modest esthetic improvement. Although most commercially available neurotoxins for esthetic use are FDA approved only for use in the upper face, the long-standing safety and efficacy profile of neurotoxins has expanded their use to many other regions. It is important to stress to patients that the result is temporary, and even with "longer acting" neurotoxins, repeat injections will be necessary to maintain the effect. It is also important to set expectations so that patients are aware of the anticipated outcomes, and modest improvements they can expect.

Clinics care points

- When injecting elevator muscles of the forehead (frontalis) always also inject the depressor muscles (corrugator, procerus) even if patients try to sway to avoid injecting those groups because they do not believe they need treatment there.
- Do not let the needle tip touch bone and then back away as is recommended by some texts. This is painful for the patient, dulls the needle, and does not improve efficacy of the treatment.
- Use the smallest bore needle possible for injection that you are able to handle without bending. This is more comfortable for the patient.
- The use of distraction devices, such a tissue vibrator, can be a useful adjunct to minimize pain

Disclosure

The author has no relevant disclosures.

Further reading

https://www.accessdata.fda.gov/drugsatfda_docs/label/2011/103000s5232lbl.pdf

https://www.accessdata.fda.gov/drugsatfda_docs/label/2016/125274s107lbl.pdf.

https://www.accessdata.fda.gov/drugsatfda_docs/label/2020/125360s078lbl.pdf.

https://www.accessdata.fda.gov/drugsatfda_docs/label/2019/761085s000lbl.pdf.

Field M, Splevins A, Picaut P, et al. AbobotulinumtoxinA (Dysport®), OnabotulinumtoxinA (Botox®), and IncobotulinumtoxinA (Xeomin®) neurotoxin content and potential implications for duration of response in patients. Toxins 2018;10(12):535.

Lee KC, Pascal AB, Halepas S, et al. What are the most commonly reported complications with cosmetic botulinum toxin type A treatments? J Oral Maxillofac Surg 2020;78(7):1190.e1–9.

Dover J, Monheit G, Greener M, et al. Botulinum toxin in aesthetic medicine: myths and realities. Dermatol Surg 2018;44(2):249–60.

Nigam PK, Nigam A. Botulinum toxin. Indian J Dermatol 2010;55(1):8–14. https://doi.org/10.4103/0019-5154.60343.

Sellin LC. The pharmacological mechanism of botulism. Trends Pharmacol Sci 1985;6:80–2.

Scaglione F. Conversion ratio between Botox®, Dysport®, and Xeomin® in clinical practice. Toxins 2016;8(3):65.

Small R. Botulinum toxin injection for facial wrinkles. Am Fam Physician 2014;90(3):168–75.

Hirsch R, Stier M. Complications and their management in cosmetic dermatology. Dermatol Clin 2009;27.

Krishtul A, Waldorf HA, Blitzer A. Complications of cosmetic botulinum toxin therapy. In: Carruthers A, editor. Botulinum toxin. Philadelphia, PA: W.B. Sanders; 2007. p. 111–21.

Niamtu J. Cosmetic facial surgery. Second Edition. Elsevier; 2018. p. 732–55.

Injectable Fillers for Lower Face Rejuvenation

Majid Rezaei, DDS, MSc*, Evan Busby, DMD, Tirbod Fattahi, DDS, MD

KEYWORDS

- Injectable filler • Lower face • Jaw line • Nonsurgical

KEY POINTS

- A well-defined jawline is an essential part of a youthful face. Gonial effacement, jowling, and retruded chin are major signs of lower face aging and comprehensive facial rejuvenation is not complete without addressing these signs.
- Nonsurgical treatment comprises the overwhelming majority of facial cosmetic procedures including lower face.
- Injectable fillers are versatile, safe, minimally invasive, with immediate results, and reversible modality for lower face rejuvenation.
- Fillers are indicated for mild to moderate facial aging. Severe volume loss, skin laxity, microgenia, and fat necks are indeed surgical cases.
- The most feared complication, though rare, is vascular compromise. The practitioner should exercise extreme caution to avoid this with a thorough understanding of anatomy, slow injection, multiple aspirations, and using a cannula.

Introduction

The lower face is an integral component of a beautiful face. Age-related changes in this region are so significant that they are often easily appreciated by patients.[1] The aging process not only includes volume loss or downward fat repositioning, but also soft tissue laxity, skin changes, and even bony resorption.[2] In the lower face, this results in sagging of the soft tissue leading to the formation of jowling, loss of an attractive well-defined jaw line, and a retruded chin. Both surgical and non-surgical options are available to reverse the aging signs; however, the popularity of non-surgical treatment has dramatically increased in last 2 decades.[3] Having a successful busy esthetic practice requires the contemporary facial surgeon to be well versed in minimally invasive techniques, have a thorough understanding of regional anatomy and physiochemical properties of the agents used.[4]

Regional anatomy

The mandible is the primary structure in lower face providing support to the overlying soft tissues. The skin and superficial fascia are retained and stabilized to the bone and deeper fascial layers by mandibular retaining ligaments and mandibular septum. This ligament arises from the anterior third of the mandible and inserts directly into the dermis.[5] Also, the subcutaneous fat in the face exists in distinct anatomic compartments.[6] There are 2 fat compartments around the mandible: superior and inferior jowl compartments.[7] These jowl compartments are located laterally to the tight mandibular ligament. As the jowl forms, its anterior extension is limited by the mandibular ligament, creating the prejowl or labio-mandibular sulcus (Fig. 1). The soft tissues are arranged differently posterior versus anterior to the prejowl sulcus.[8] Posterior to the sulcus, skin, subcutaneous fat, platysma, deep fat, parotido-masseteric fascia, masseter muscle, and periosteum of the mandible form the soft tissue thickness. Anterior to the sulcus, however, skin and subcutaneous fat lay over the expression muscles (depressor anguli oris, platysma, depressor labia inferioris, and mentalis), deep fat, and periosteum (Fig. 2).

Injectable fillers

Almost all types of fillers including Hyaluronic Acid (HA), Poly-L-Lactic Acid (PLLA), Calcium hydroxyapatite, and Poly-Methyl-Methacrylate (PMMA) could be used in lower face.[4] HA fillers simply add more volume to facial soft tissues and are most popular. PLLA actively stimulates the body reaction with subsequent fibroplasia. The mechanism of action of PMMA and calcium hydroxyapatite is combination of both.[9] Fillers are usually designed to be injected at a certain tissue level. However, experienced practitioners frequently use fillers in multiple tissue planes in order to achieve the optimal results and sometimes even utilize different types of filler for the same injection site.[10] The thinner (less viscous) fillers with small particle sizes are designed for superficial skin layers, though the thicker fillers with relatively larger particles are intended to use in deeper tissue planes (deep skin, subcutaneous, or periosteal layers). Injecting viscous or particulate filler too superficially may result in irregularities or could be visible through the skin. In contrast, placing a thin filler in the deep tissue planes could lead to premature resorption. G prime

Department of Oral and Maxillofacial Surgery, College of Medicine, University of Florida Health, Jacksonville, FL, USA
* Corresponding author. 653 8th Street West, Jacksonville, FL 32209.
E-mail address: majid.rezaei@jax.ufl.edu

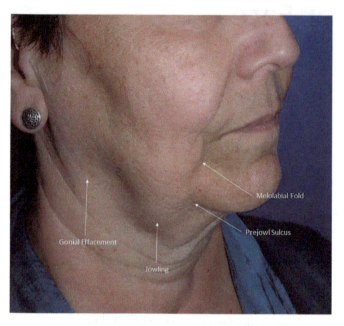

Fig. 1 Age-related changes in lower face.

is another measurement of fillers which indicates hardness and ability to cause tissue projection.[10] While some clinicians prefer high G prime HA fillers, the others like calcium hydroxyapatite or PLLA in both prejowl and chin regions. Regardless, these fillers should be placed deep into the tissues, for example, supra-periosteal. (the authors need to add a

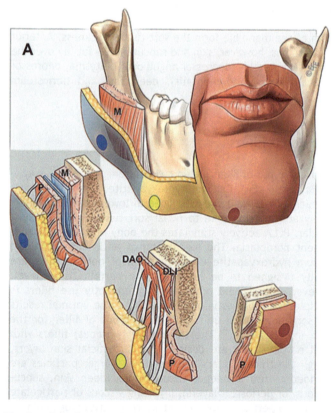

Fig. 2 Soft tissue arrangement anterior and posterior to the prejowl sulcus. (*Reprinted with permission from* Springer: Minelli, L., Yang, HM., van der Lei, B. et al. The Surgical Anatomy of the Jowl and the Mandibular Ligament Reassessed. Aesth Plast Surg 47, 170–180 (2023))

figure to show the superficial vs deep layers). In addition, it is a common practice to treat the melomental area with concurrent neuromodulation.

Clinical evaluation

The esthetic goal in lower face rejuvenation is to straighten the jawline, to elevate the jowls in a posterosuperior direction,[11] and to restore a well-defined pleasant chin and angle of the jaw.

In general, injectables are best indicated for mild to moderate imperfections. Patients with severe contour or volume loss, skin laxity and redundancy, or microgenia are probably better suited with surgical options. It is imperative to carefully listen to the patient and understand their complaints and concerns. In those who are considered medically high risk or are adamant against surgery, limitations of injectable treatment and realistic expectations should be discussed (Fig. 3).

Patients with fat atrophy or descending jowling with a slim neck would benefit most from injectables and would see the results instantly. On the contrary, fillers would not make a visible change in patients with excess fat in neck and submental areas. Therefore, patient selection is very important to be able to achieve their certain goals.

As with other facial cosmetic procedures, the face must be evaluated as a whole. Assessment of facial thirds and vertical fifths is the basis of any facial analysis and helps the clinician localize imbalances and asymmetries. Clinical evaluation must be completed at rest and animation while patient is in upright position, with Frankfurt horizontal line parallel to the ground. Photographs are obtained in the frontal, profile and three-fourth views. Attention is then given to the prominence of the mandibular angle, jawline, chin projection and length, jowling, and prejowl sulcus. The anatomic differences between males and females should be taken into account. In general, males have stronger jaw, more prominent angle and chin compared to females. In frontal view, bigonial and bizygomatic distances are equal in males. However, a youthful female face is characterized by the inverted "triangle of youth," with a bizygomatic distance wider than the bigonial distance.[2] (Fig. 4) There are different methods to define the ideal chin position in frontal and sagittal planes and in depths description of these methods are beyond the scope of this article. Some simple analyses based on soft tissue measurements are briefly explained here. In profile view chin projection is primarily related to the nose and the lips. Soft tissue chin is 2 to 6 mm behind a perpendicular line drawn from the subnasale.[12] Alternatively, chin projection could be assessed with regards to a perpendicular line from soft tissue nasion. An ideal chin is located on, or falls just short of, this line.[13] The clinicians should pay special attention to male patients with deficient chin as they may camouflage their retruded chin with beards (Fig. 5). The height of the chin must be seen in the context of lower facial height. The upper lip height (distance from the subnasale to the upper lip stomion) should be a half of the distance from stomion to the menton.[12] Finally, the transverse width of the chin in females is equal to the intercanthal distance, whereas it spans the distance between the right and left oral commissures in males.[13] (Fig. 6).

Technique

This section covers the common techniques for rejuvenation of lower face with injectables. However, it is noteworthy that

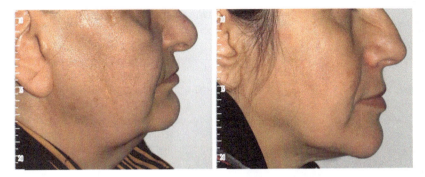

Fig. 3 Patients with severe skin laxity and redundancy, and microgenia (left) are surgical candidate. In contrast, patients with mild-moderate imperfections and a slim neck (right) could be efficiently treated with injectables.

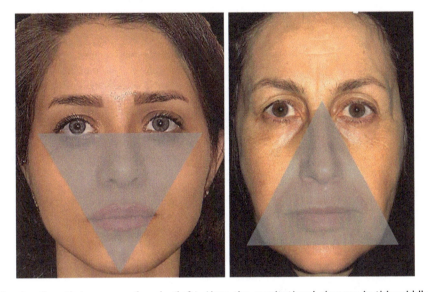

Fig. 4 Inverted triangle of youth in a young female (left). Note the gravitational changes in this middle age female (right).

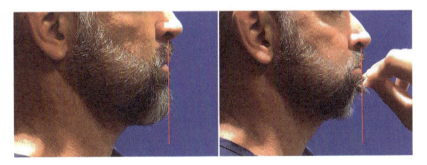

Fig. 5 Camouflage of the retruded chin in a male patient with retrogenia.

volume loss in the midface and upper face leads to skin ptosis in lower face. Therefore, to counteract this effect, the best approach begins with addressing the midface and upper face volume loss and laxity. Restoring volume of the cheeks helps alleviate the prominence of nasolabial folds and marionette lines.

Although most fillers contain lidocaine in their formulations, use of topical anesthetic is highly recommended on all patients. Mental nerve blocks through intra-oral mucosa provide excellent anesthesia and comfort when addressing chin and prejowl regions.

Prior to the injection, the designated injection sites must be meticulously prepared using an alcohol pad. Ensure all makeups are completely removed, as penetration of microbial biofilm or makeup particles into the skin during injection may cause inflammation, or infection.

Another controversial issue is using needles versus cannula. Many believe needles provide the most precise injection control. Also, needles penetrate more easily through previous surgical sites and scar tissues compared to cannula. However, some feel that cannula may be safer than needles with less chance of inadvertent intra-vascular injections as well as causing less bruising.

Some clinicians prefer supine position for injection, while others advise a semi-supine or sitting position as the supine position may mask imperfections such as nasolabial or

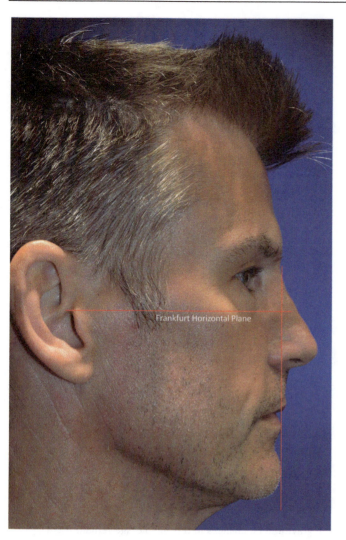

Fig. 6 An ideal chin is located on, or fall just short of a perpendicular line drawn from soft tissue nasion. Note the Frankfurt Horizontal plane is parallel to the ground.

Mandibular angle

- Thoroughly clean the facial skin with an antiseptic solution. Ensure coverage extends below the jawline and onto the preauricular region.
- Localize the tip of the mandibular angle. It is always helpful to draw markings over the intended areas to be augmented. Depending on your global facial measurements and patient desires, augmentation could include only the angle, or inferior mandible and posterior ramus borders as well (Fig. 7).
- Some injectors place the filler only in subcutaneous layer, while other recommend submasseteric injection for the angle area combined with subcutaneous injection along the inferior and posterior borders.
- If the angle of mandible is the only treatment area in lower face, the injection site is right on top of the deficient angle (Fig. 8). If you are addressing both the angle and jowling regions, 1 cm posterior to the jowling could be your entrance point for both areas. Be mindful of facial vessels which are typically located 3 cm anterior to the mandibular angle (Fig. 9). Either anterograde or retrograde injection method could be utilized. Begin with small depots (0.1–0.2 mL) in the angle area. Re-evaluate facial proportions before adding more fillers. Total volume injected varies from patient to patient, average being 1.5 mL per side, but can be more if needed (Fig. 10).
- Upon completion of the filler injection, apply digital massage to mold the fillers along the jaw line and posterior ramus border.

Chin

- Chin augmentation frequently requires injections into multiple layers.
- It is sometimes necessary to utilize a neuromodulator 10 to 14 days prior to filler injection, in order to relax an overactive mentalis muscles, thus increasing the treatment longevity.
- Tracing a chin implant over the skin could provide an excellent easy template for injection.[10]
- Employ bilateral mental nerve block, as multi-layer filler injection could be painful.
- Entrance point could be slightly posterior to the melolabial groove (prejowl sulcus) on either side (Fig. 11).

melomental folds. Either position could be used as long as the clinician evaluates the interim or final results in sitting position.

Last but not the least, always aspirate multiple times during injection, whether you are using needle or cannula. To minimize the risk of complications, it is advisable to employ a technique involving low-pressure and slow injections of small volumes.[11]

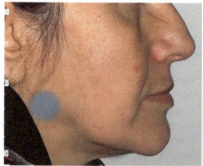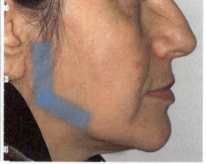

Fig. 7 The tip of the mandibular angle (blue circle in left image). Inferior mandible and posterior ramus borders are also accessible via the same entrance point (Right).

Injectable Fillers for Lower Face Rejuvenation

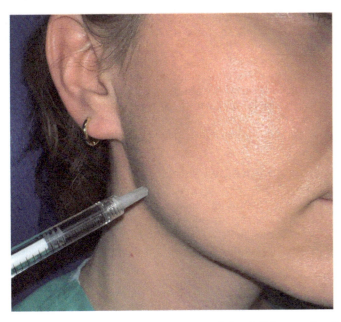

Fig. 8 The injection site right on top of the deficient angle of mandible.

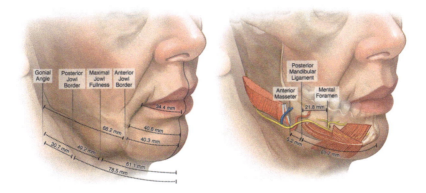

Fig. 9 Important anatomic structures and their relationship to surface skin topography. (*Reprinted with permission from* Springer: Minelli, L., Yang, HM., van der Lei, B. et al. The Surgical Anatomy of the Jowl and the Mandibular Ligament Reassessed. Aesth Plast Surg 47, 170–180 (2023))

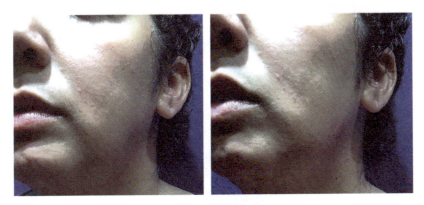

Fig. 10 Mandibuiolar angle augmentation with Hyaluronic Acid filler. Pretreatment (left). Post-treatment (Right).

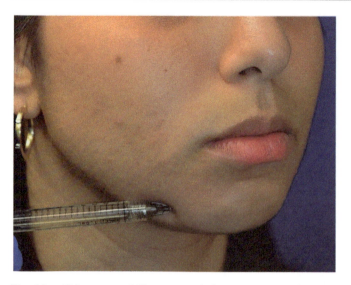

Fig. 11 Chin area could be accessed via an entrance point at or slightly posterior to pre-jowl sulcus.

- The soft tissue chin including mentalis muscle is pinched and elevated so submuscular injection is facilitated. 0.1 mL of the filler is injected supra-periosteally in the midline. On withdrawal, 2 to 3 smaller supra-periosteal depots are placed lateral to the midline injection on both sides to tapering toward the prejowl sulcus. This must be repeated in muscular layer, starting from midline and tapering laterally. Subcutaneous injections could be reserved for final contouring (Fig. 12).

Jowling and prejowl sulcus

- Although almost any commercially available filler can be used in this region, more viscous with higher G prime filler (such as calcium hydroxyapatite or a Juvéderm Voluma) is preferred for injections directly along the bony margin.
- Local anesthesia via intra-oral mental nerve block is recommended
- Entrance point could be lateral to the jowling, especially if the angle and jawline is also planned for injection. In

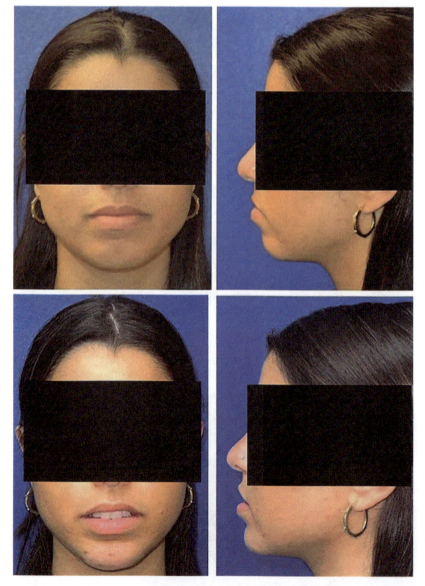

Fig. 12 Chin contouring with 2 mL of Hyaluronic Acid filler. Pre-treatment (upper right and left). Post-treatment (lower right and left).

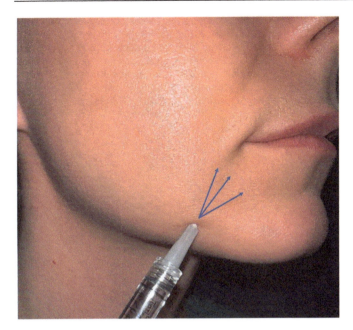

Fig. 13 Fanning technique for augmentation of marionette line.

case the prejowl sulcus is the only intended site, filler could be injected perpendicularly directly onto the bone.
- Melomental fold also known as marionette line could be addressed through the same entry point for prejowl sulcus. However, the filler should be placed in the deep dermal plane versus the supra-periosteal plane in prejowl sulcus area. Small aliquots are injected in retrograde (or anterograde) and fanning fashion (Fig. 13).
- Again, gentle massage is mandatory to smoothen the injected area and achieve an even distribution of the filler material.
- Downward pull from depressor anguli oris muscle plays a major role in persistent marionette lines. Therefore, many advocate partial paralysis of this muscle by administering 2 to 4 units of neurotoxins in mid-portion of the muscle. It could be done at the same time of filler injection or sequentially in 2 different appointments. The injection site for neurotoxin is half way between the oral commissure and prejowl sulcus (inferior jawline).

Complications

Lower face rejuvenation with injectable fillers, like other part of the face, is usually safe and uneventful. Uncommon occasions of edema, erythema, bruising, or irritation are often mild, transient, and self-limiting. Foreign body granuloma formations (especially with intra-muscular injections) and inadvertent intra-parotid injection with subsequent parotitis are rare, though a cosmetic injector should be mindful of. The most severe and feared complication is indeed vascular compromise due to either unintended intravascular injection or hydrostatic collapse as a result of impending pressure of a filler materials surrounding the vessel. Early signs of ischemia include pallor and blanching, unexpected and unexplainable pain during the injection or shortly after. If left untreated, this may lead to blue discoloration and eventually tissue necrosis. Subcutaneous layer in lower face is relatively free of major vasculature. Facial artery and vein are closest to surface at the inferior border of mandible. The blunt cannulae are therefore recommended in higher risk areas of vascular compromise as they are less likely to injure blood vessels. Nevertheless, the best treatment is prevention. A good knowledge of anatomy, aspiration prior to and during injection, slow and low pressure injection, and injection on withdrawal are the best preventive measures.

In case the injector recognizes the ischemic signs, he/she must stop the procedure immediately, apply warm compression with massage. Local administration of hyaluronidase around the suspected occluded or embolized vessel (500–1000 units) has also been recommended. The use of aspirin, topical nitroglycerin, or low molecular weight heparin has also been reported, even though their application is more controversial.

Clinics care points

- Injectable fillers are quite easy tools for lower facial rejuvenation. However, the the clinician must be knowledgable about the filler composition and facial anatomy to prevent serious complications.
- It is a prudent strategy, for a novice injector or a new filler patient, to start with resorbable fillers such as HA, since the undesirable outcomes or complications could be more easily reversed and managed.
- Multi-layer injection provides the most desirable and durable results. The deeper plane filler adds the necessary bulk and projection, while the superficial injection brings about topographic details, sharp edges and line angles.
- Vascular compromise and soft tissue loss following filler injection are exceedingly rare in lower face. Early recognition, halting the procedure, and initiating the emergency treatement would decrease the risk of permanent deficit.

Disclosure

Authors have no relevant conflict of interest with this article.

References

1. Reece EM, Rohrich RJ. The aesthetic jaw line: management of the aging jowl. Aesthetic Surg J 2008;28(6):668–74.
2. Vazirnia A, Braz A, Fabi SG. Nonsurgical jawline rejuvenation using injectable fillers. J Cosmet Dermatol 2020;19(8):1940–7.
3. Hari-Raj A, Spataro EA. Evidence-based medicine for nonsurgical facial rejuvenation. Facial Plast Surg 2023;39(3):230–6.
4. Braz A, Humphrey S, Weinkle S, et al. Lower face: clinical anatomy and regional approaches with injectable fillers. Plast Reconstr Surg 2015;136(5 Suppl):235S–57S.
5. Kang MS, Kang HG, Nam YS, et al. Detailed anatomy of the retaining ligaments of the mandible for facial rejuvenation. J Cranio-Maxillo-Fac Surg 2016;44(9):1126–30.
6. Rohrich RJ, Pessa JE. The fat compartments of the face: anatomy and clinical implications for cosmetic surgery. Plast Reconstr Surg 2007;119(7):2219–27.
7. Reece EM, Pessa JE, Rohrich RJ. The mandibular septum: anatomical observations of the jowls in aging-implications for facial rejuvenation. Plast Reconstr Surg 2008;121(4):1414–20.
8. Braz A, Eduardo CCP. Reshaping the lower face using injectable fillers. Indian J Plast Surg 2020;53(2):207–18.

9. Fitzgerald R, Graivier MH, Kane M, et al. Appropriate selection and application of nonsurgical facial rejuvenation agents and procedures: panel consensus recommendations. Aesthet Surg J 2010;30(Suppl):36S–45S.
10. Niamtu JWJ, Barbarino S, Rivikin A, et al. Injectable fillers and surgical lip lift. In: *Cosmetic facial surgery*. 3 edition. Philadelphia, PA: Elsevier; 2022. p. 678–770.
11. Parsa KM, Somenek M. Nonsurgical jaw contouring: a multi-faceted approach. Clin Plast Surg 2023;50(3):489–96.
12. Epker B. Evaluation of the face, In: Fonseca R., Oral and Maxillofacial Surgery, Vol.3, 2nd edition, 2008, Saunders; St. Louis, MO, 4.
13. Vanaman Wilson MJ, Jones IT, Butterwick K, et al. Role of nonsurgical chin augmentation in full face rejuvenation: a review and our experience. Dermatol Surg 2018;44(7):985–93.

Perioral Filler Augmentation

Faisal A. Quereshy, MD, DDS, George F. Schieder IV, DMD*

KEYWORDS

- Perioral filler • Lip filler • Perioral vertical lip rhytids • Marionette lines • Nasolabial folds

KEY POINTS

- Perioral tissues present some of the first signs of the aging face, and thus, perioral fillers are oftentimes the first cosmetic procedures requested by patients.
- Perioral fillers provide a temporary means of augmenting volume and softening common lines of the face.
- Injections in the perioral area can include the lips, nasolabial folds, philtral columns, vertical lip rhytids (perioral "smoker lines"), oral commissures, melomental folds (marionette lines), mentolabial folds, and nasolabial folds.
- Technique of perioral filler injection depends on the region, product, and desired augmentation.

Introduction

Perioral tissues, similar to all tissues, undergo aging due to decreased proliferative capacity, accumulating cellular damage, and inherited genetic predispositions. These changes can be exacerbated by extrinsic factors such as sun exposure, tobacco use, and mechanical stress. Perioral augmentation can help mask many age-related changes of the face. The presence of nasolabial folds is one of the earliest esthetic complaints made by patients (Fig. 1A). Nasolabial folds continue to deepen with age (see Fig. 1B). Over time, lip volume diminishes and the vermillion border loses definition. Even young patients without physical signs of aging seek lip filler for an esthetic boost. A pronounced cupid's bow with defined *philtral columns* is a common display of youthful lips. Conversely, thin lips result in deepened oral commissures, which can give patients a frowning look at rest. Melolabial folds, commonly called "marionette lines," are resting lines from the oral commissures extending inferiorly, which, along with nasolabial folds, accentuate jowling. The mentolabial fold is a horizontal line that can present between the lower lip and chin as the lip volume thins and the chin begins to sag. Perioral vertical rhytids are typically an esthetic complaint of the elderly face (see Fig. 1C). These are colloquially called "smoker lines" due to the earlier presentation caused by repetitive pursing of the orbicularis oris during smoking. With age, fine lines can develop anywhere on the face from decades of muscular movement and sun exposure.

Surgical technique

Preoperative Planning

Although each filler product has different properties, recommendations can differ among injectors depending on experience and availability of product. Ultimately, choice of filler is a personal choice that can be altered for each clinical scenario. Important properties to consider include firmness (G′), cohesivity (resistance to spread), and water affinity. An overly simplified spectrum exists—on one end are low-density, low G′ fillers commonly described as "silky, smooth, thin, flowable" such as Juvederm Volbella, Restylane Refyne or Silk, and Revance RHA Redensity. On the other end are high-density, high G′ fillers commonly described as "hard, dense, solid, bulky" such as Juvederm Voluma, Restylane Lyft, and Revance RHA 4. A useful resource regarding filler choice will be the producer's websites because many manufacturers market certain filler products for certain regions of the face.

Management of expectations is the most important step in cosmetic procedures. In all cases, the injector should review expectations with the patient, using both preop photographs and a mirror.

As part of expectation management, the patient should be counseled to expect the need for "touch-ups," rather than expecting a perfect result after a single appointment (Fig. 2). This may not be needed but better to set the expectation and not need it, rather than confront a patient who was expecting one appointment for perfection. Patients should be counseled about the degree of edema, erythema, and ecchymosis that can present in the perioral areas following injections. Especially for injections to the lip, the true cosmetic result will be less than the immediate post-injection appearance. Patients commonly seek out filler before important events such as weddings, birthdays, and vacations. Given the possibility of edema and ecchymosis following injections, we recommend filler augmentations be delayed in such cases.

Prep and Patient Positioning

Before injecting, the patient's skin is cleaned using standard alcohol wipes. Novice practitioners may find a marking pencil helpful for planning and discussing expectations with the patient. Local anesthesia for filler injections can range from no anesthesia to regional nerve blocks. Whether additional anesthesia is planned or not, ice packs applied to the face are recommended to

Department of Oral & Maxillofacial Surgery, Case Western Reserve University, 9601 Chester Avenue, Cleveland, OH 44106, USA
* Corresponding author.
E-mail address: GeorgeSchieder@me.com

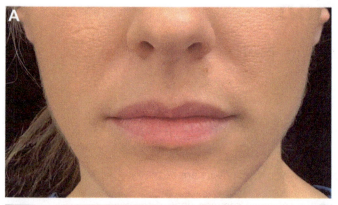
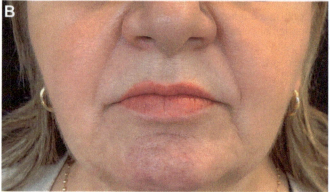
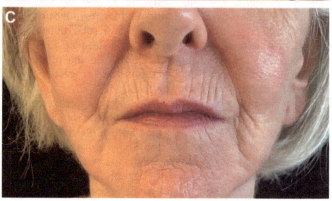

Fig. 1 (*A*) This 31-year-old woman presented with early perioral age changes of the nasolabial folds. (*B*) Compare this to a 56-year-old woman with deepening of the nasolabial folds and marionette lines. (*C*) Compare this to a 71-year-old woman presenting with deep nasolabial folds, marionette lines, thinning skin, thinning lips, and several perioral vertical rhytids.

reduce swelling and also give the benefit of temporary skin anesthesia. Many filler products contain lidocaine, and thus will anesthetize locally as injections progress. Many providers find topical anesthetics useful, which are applied up to 60 minutes before injections. Complete anesthesia of the perioral region can be easily achieved with bilateral mental nerve (Fig. 3) and infraorbital nerve (Fig. 4) blocks. Although this approach is very effective, some patients are uncomfortable with the profound degree of anesthesia that results in temporary drooling, inability to eat, and loss of facial sensation for the duration of the anesthetic. Positioning of the patient for perioral augmentation is always in the upright position. The supine position changes the vector of gravity on tissues, which is oftentimes what perioral filler is attempting to overcome or mask. The injector should inject and observe progress from multiple angles.

Lip Filler

The technique for lip filler augmentation is based on the desired change in shape. The upper lip can be thought of as 3 tubercles with an "M"-shaped border, and the lower lip is thought of as 2 tubercles with a "U"-shaped border as shown in Fig. 5. The lips should not be filled as one continuous unit of even density.

Increased volume of the lips is accomplished by injecting product into the orbicularis oris muscle. The needle is inserted near the vermillion border (Fig. 6), advanced, and product is injected as the needle is withdrawn. Typically in younger patients, the regions of the lips lateral to the ala of the nose are not injected to avoid "sausaging" of the lip (Fig. 7); however, older patients with deepened commissures (Fig. 8) often benefit from injections extending to the commissure.

For the lower lip, a subtle midline cleavage is oftentimes desired to accentuate the bilateral pillars of bulk and prevent one long "tube" look. This can be achieved by inserting dental floss between the mandibular midline contact and holding the floss vertically against the lower lip during injections and molding (Fig. 9).

If the intended change in shape is increased vertical height of the lip, the needle can be inserted vertically from the vermillion border. Product is then threaded upward on withdrawal as shown in Fig. 10.

Following injections, petroleum jelly is placed on the lips and a gentle massage is carried out to smoothen the product. This can be achieved by gently pinching the lip from the extraoral and intraoral sides and molding of the product (Fig. 11). The less dense fillers are especially amenable to massage to achieve a result without lumps or asymmetries.

Especially in the elderly face, patients may seek increased definition of the vermillion border specifically. To achieve this, the needle is inserted horizontally following the vermillion border.

However, instead of injecting deeper in the muscularis, the product is deposited more superficially to give a defined, accented vermillion border. Fig. 12 demonstrates the result for a patient who specifically requested a more pronounced vermillion border. This defined border is commonly lost in middle age.

An esthetic subnasal region depends on a pair of well-defined columella and vermillion border, giving rise to a pronounced cupid's bow and philtrum. To define the columella, the needle is inserted at the peak of the cupid's bow on either side and advanced to the base of the nose, following the natural course of the pillars (Fig. 13). Product is injected on withdrawal. It is essential to follow a natural angle of the philtral columns, which are usually slightly diverging from the subnasale to the vermillion border, ending in the bilateral peaks of the cupid's bow (Fig. 14). Parallel or asymmetrically diverging columns will result in an unesthetic infranasal region.

Many first-time patients request low volumes due to concerns of a "fake look" from too much filler. Generally, 0.5 mL or less to the lips will have virtually no perceivable effect once swelling has resolved (Fig. 15). A reasonable starting volume for virgin lips is around 1.0 mL (1 syringe), which should provide a noticeable effect to the patient without concern for excess. Too much volume into virgin lips increases the risk of filler migration into the surrounding skin, giving the dreaded "duck lip" appearance.

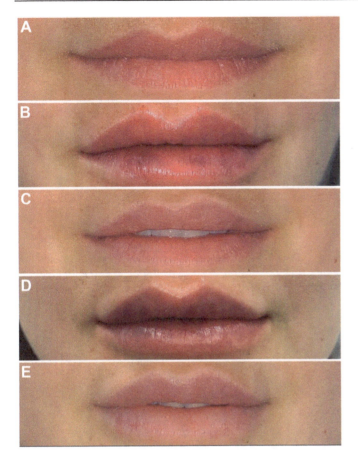

Fig. 2 (*A*) A 30-year-old woman's preop photo. This patient's lips seemed symmetric immediately after injections (*B*), however, note the asymmetry of the upper lip following resolution of swelling (*C*). Additional filler was placed (*D*) to achieve a more symmetric final result (*E*).

Perioral Vertical Rhytid Filler

Perioral "smoker lines" are often extremely fine. Rather than injecting product linearly on withdrawal similar to many other filler injection techniques, the approach to vertical lip rhytids

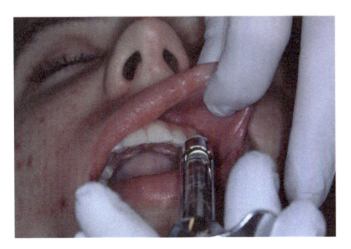

Fig. 3 Complete anesthesia of the perioral region can be easily achieved with bilateral mental nerve and infraorbital nerve blocks. To achieve an infraorbital nerve block, a long 27-gauge needle is inserted in the maxillary vestibule apical to the canine tooth or first premolar and advanced superiorly to the infraorbital region.

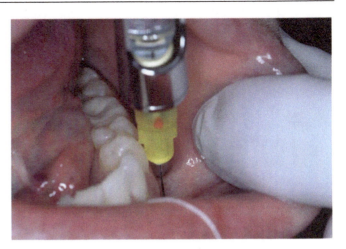

Fig. 4 To achieve a mental nerve block, the needle enters at the mandibular vestibule near the first and second premolar, and the needle is advanced inferiorly to the area of the mental foramen.

should be small boluses that are massaged through the lines. As shown in Fig. 16, the needle is inserted near the vermillion border, advanced, and a very small bolus is injected superficially in the center of the line. The product is then massaged to fill the fine rhytid. For this reason, the lowest density fillers are needed such as Juvederm Volbella or Restylane Silk. Some authors also recommend creating perpendicular threads deeper under the vertical lines to create a lattice to bulk the thin tissue.

Fine lines of the face can be tenacious. A mistake would be aggressive deposition of product that would leave the tissue distorted. For many perioral fillers, it is wise to treat half of the face and demonstrate the difference to the patient, as in Fig. 17. As for all perioral filler, edema begins almost immediately and will obscure the final look. Small amounts of filler over multiple appointments can oftentimes be the best option for fine lines to avoid overfilling and distortion of tissues

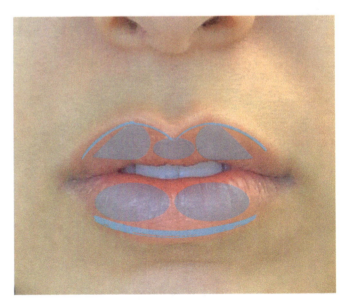

Fig. 5 Overlay of the lips displaying the areas of anatomic bulk and curved borders. The upper lip can be thought of as 3 tubercles with an "M"-shaped border, and the lower lip is thought of as 2 tubercles with a "U"-shaped border.

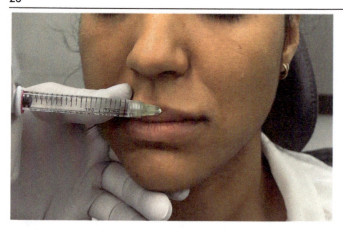

Fig. 6 The needle is inserted horizontally near the vermillion border and advanced to its destination, keeping in mind the natural shape of the lip.

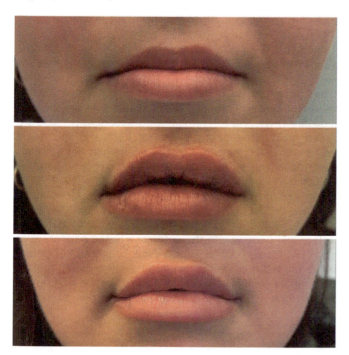

Fig. 7 This younger patient was satisfied with her result but note the lateral bulk of the top lip, which can result from extending the filler too far laterally.

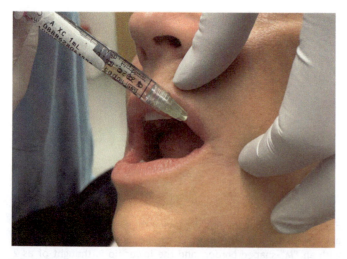

Fig. 8 Advancing the needle to the oral commissure of this patient is indicated due to the lack of lip volume and deepened commissure, although this is typically avoided in younger patients.

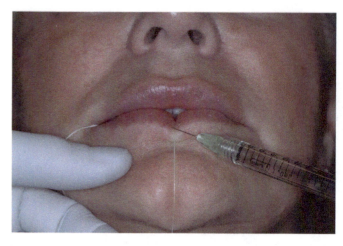

Fig. 9 Dental floss inserted between the mandibular midline contact is held firmly on the midline during injection to create a final result respecting the natural anatomy.

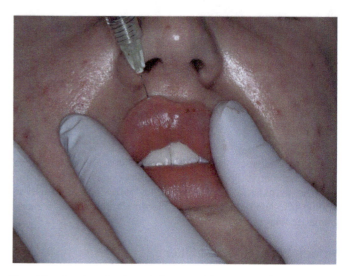

Fig. 10 Product is threaded upward in a vertical direction to achieve an increased vertical height of the lip.

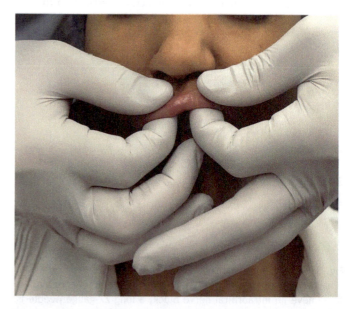

Fig. 11 The product is smoothened by gently massaging the lip from both the extraoral and intraoral sides.

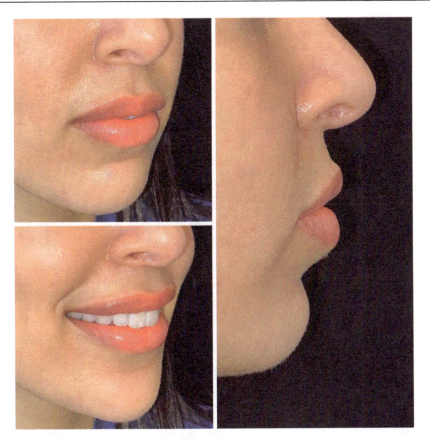

Fig. 12 More superficial injections along the vermillion border provided this patient with her desired result of a more pronounced border.

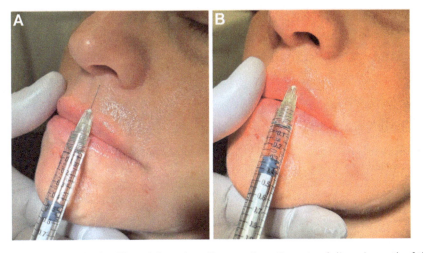

Fig. 13 (A) Lining up the path of the needle for filler of the columella, note how the natural diverging path of the columella is respected. (B) The needle is inserted at the peak of the cupid's bow and advanced. Product is injected on withdrawal.

(Fig. 18). Lip filler before vertical rhytid injections improves the result because volume in the upper lip can reduce the appearance of vertical lip rhytids, even before direct injection of the lines themselves.

Nasolabial Fold Filler

Nasolabial filler follows the nasolabial fold from the ala of the nose to the oral commissure.

Thin product will displace, while thick product may produce a bulky, static look. Medium density products such as Juvederm Ultra or Juvederm Vollure work well for nasolabial folds. Nasolabial folds can accept a surprising amount of filler to achieve a noticeable effect, and due to the cost of filler, patients should be consented for multiple syringes of filler. Oftentimes, at least 1.0 mL is needed per side, and in elderly patients, the folds can accept 3.0 mL or more. The depth of nasolabial fold filler can be placed dermal or deep, with more severe nasolabial folds often requiring both levels of placement for optimal effect.

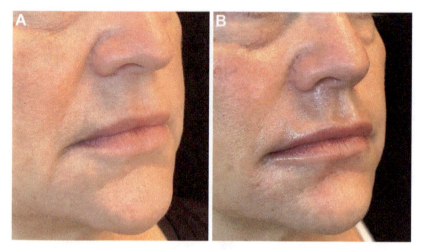

Fig. 14 (A) Preop of a patient complaining of poorly defined lips. (B) Immediate postop showing how the columella filler can produce a more pronounced philtrum.

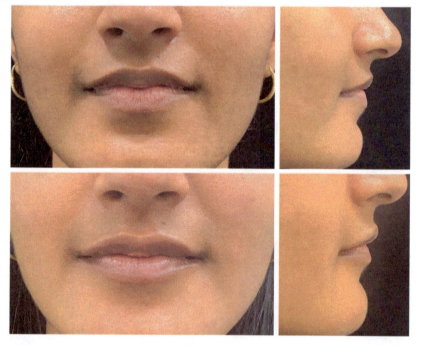

Fig. 15 This young patient received ~0.6 mL of Juvederm Volbella XC spread between the upper and lower lip, giving her a very subtle bump in volume. Any less filler would have likely produced no perceptible difference.

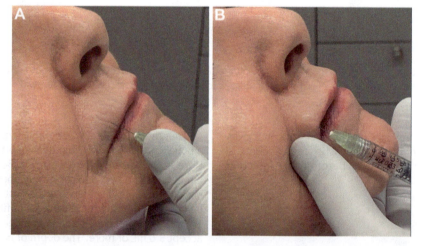

Fig. 16 (A) The needle held over the intended path of insertion, (B) the needle is inserted, "tented" to test depth, and a small aliquot is placed.

Perioral Filler Augmentation

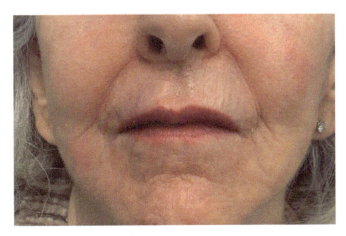

Fig. 17 A 70-year-old patient with filler injected to the right side perioral vertical rhytids before treating the left. Note the softened appearance of the vertical *lines*. As for all perioral filler, edema begins almost immediately.

Pulling of the nasolabial fold from the oral commissure straightens the fold, allowing for straight injection of product (Fig. 19A). Measuring the length of the needle against the skin will demonstrate the entry point for injection to reach the desired location (see Fig. 19B). The needle is advanced, and then the product is injected linearly on withdrawal (see Fig. 19C). Injections are started at the ala of the nose and carried sequentially inferiorly to the oral commissure (see Fig. 19D). Filler is generally injected medial/inferior to the fold (Fig. 20) because lateral/superior injection can accentuate the descending tissue of the cheek. Small threads of filler perpendicular to the fold can also soften the depth of the fold. As with all techniques, the injected filler is massaged smooth (Fig. 21).

Marionette Line Filler

Marionette line filler follows the same principles as nasolabial fold filler—the skin is pulled taught to produce a linear fold, and product is placed sequentially from the oral commissure (Fig. 22). Just as for nasolabial folds, filler can be injected in small lines perpendicular to the fold to soften the final result. When treating marionette lines, filler is commonly fanned at the lateral lip near the oral commissure to soften the depth of deep commissures that can accentuate the marionette line (Fig. 23). The filler is smoothed (Fig. 24), and the patient can be shown the treated side before continuing on the contralateral side (Fig. 25).

Mentolabial Filler

Mentolabial lines are horizontal skin creases inferior to the lower lip. Following similar principles to other perioral fillers, the needle is advanced along the dermal layer and injected on withdrawal, followed by massage (Fig. 26).

Postoperative care

- The injection sites should immediately receive cold to reduce edema and bruising.
- Advise patients to avoid heavy exercise following injections.

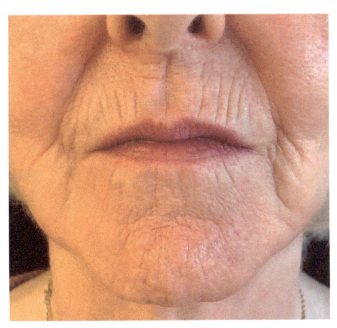

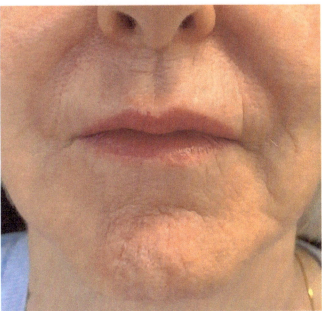

Fig. 18 Before and after photos following multiple visits for treatment of vertical lip rhytids. This patient also received filler to the upper lip to help improve the look of the vertical *lines*.

- Makeup is avoided for 48 hours to prevent irritation at the puncture sites.
- Reassurance is important in the recovery period because patients will have a more volumized look than the final result.

Potential complications

Complications of filler injection are detailed in a later article of this text. However, it is worth noting that the lips are especially prone to swelling and bruising following needle puncture (Fig. 27). Cold, applied immediately before and post-procedure, is the patient's best defense against edema and ecchymosis. Similar to all surgical postop edema, swelling usually peaks in 3 to 5 days before gradually tapering. A tapering steroid dose can

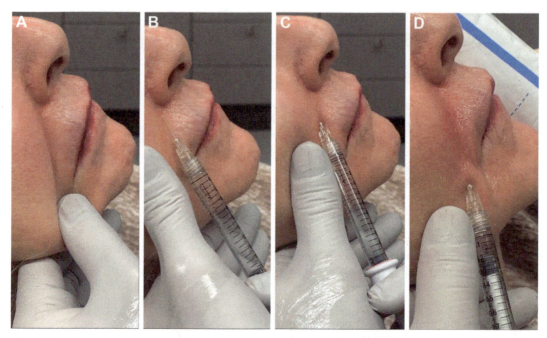

Fig. 19 (A) Stretching of the skin to produce a straight nasolabial fold for injection, (B) lining up the needle to the intended target area, (C) insertion and injection, and (D) continuing stepwise inferiorly along the fold.

be considered in certain cases (Fig. 28). Injections to the lip can stimulate eruptions of recurrent herpes simplex virus, so patients with known recurrent herpes can be placed on the appropriate antivirals. As shown in Fig. 29, a combination of HA fillers for perioral augmentation often gives the best result.

Similar to all areas of the face, the local vasculature of the perioral region presents a vascular occlusion risk. Most relevant to perioral injections are the following.

- The lips are supplied by the superior labial and inferior labial arteries branching from the facial artery. Based on cadaveric studies, these arteries are typically found in the posterior/mucosal half of the lip; thus, injections to the lips in the orbicularis oris should be kept in the anterior/skin half.
- The nasolabial fold parallels the course of the facial artery because it travels superiorly from the mandibular border to the lateral nasal region where it becomes the angular artery. Caution is recommended if injecting deep near the ala.

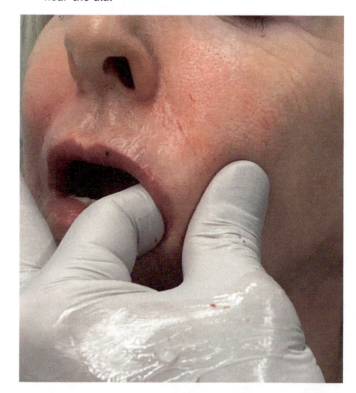

Fig. 20 Injection of the nasolabial fold showing the placement of product slightly inferior to the fold.

Fig. 21 Massage of the injected filler is completed with an index finger inside the oral cavity and the thumb on the skin. Note the petroleum jelly placed on the glove to be used on the skin during massage.

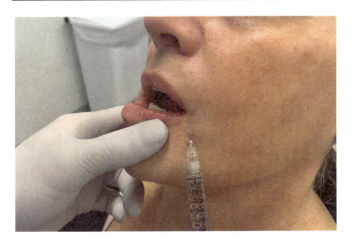

Fig. 22 Injection technique for the marionette *line*, beginning at the oral commissure.

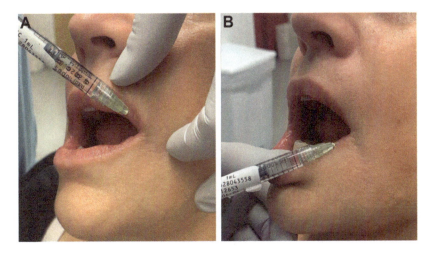

Fig. 23 Fanning injection of filler at the lateral commissure from the upper (*A*) and lower lip (*B*) to soften the marionette line.

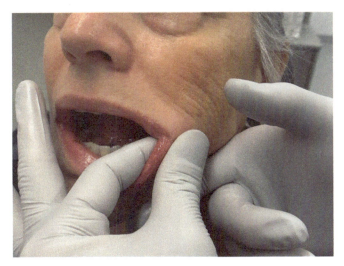

Fig. 24 Massage of the marionette line filler after injection, rolling the product from both the intraoral and extraoral sides.

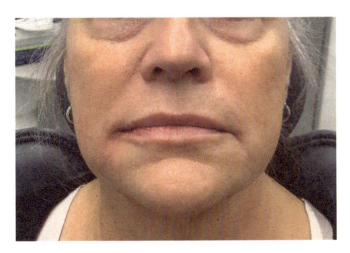

Fig. 25 Intraoperative photo demonstrating a treated right marionette *line* vs an untreated left—note the softened *line* as well as the reduced depth of the oral commissure, reducing the downturned "frowning" look of the patient at rest.

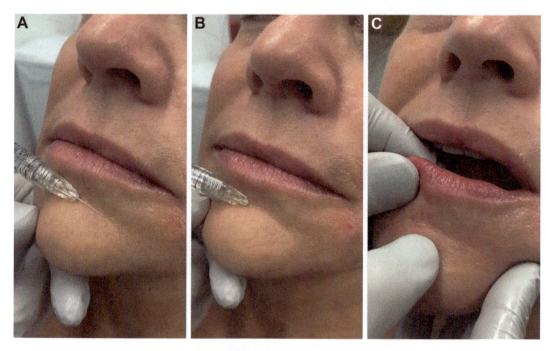

Fig. 26 (A) The needle is lined up to the mentolabial fold, (B) advanced along the dermal layer and injected on withdrawal, followed by massage (C).

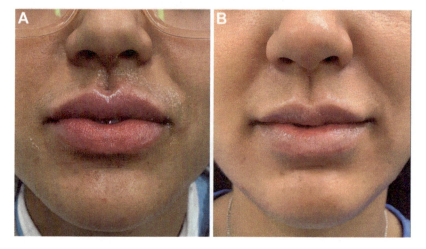

Fig. 27 (A) Showing postinjection swelling in a female patient receiving lip filler compared with (B) the eventual result after 2 weeks.

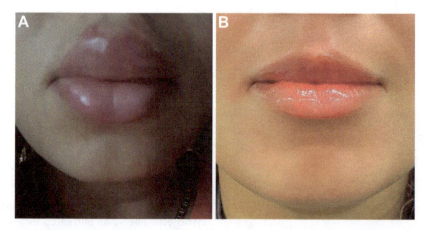

Fig. 28 (A) This home photograph on the left was taken by a patient hours after lip filler. (B) The patient was started on a tapering steroid dose, which resulted in rapid improvement.

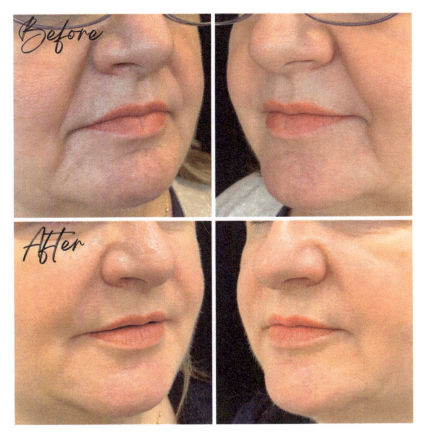

Fig. 29 Results of a combination of HA fillers for perioral augmentation.

Clinics care points

- Many first-time cosmetic patients seek out filler to the lips or nasolabial folds as their first cosmetic procedure; thus, management of expectations is critical for these patients with no previous filler experience!
- Because of the degree of edema from lip injections, postop symmetry does not always result in final symmetry. Patients should be counseled to expect the need for "touch ups."
- Typically, the denser the filler, the deeper it is injected. Perioral regions often require less-dense filler that is injected more superficially into the dermis beneath the line being treated, although for deep folds, layering and perpendicular threading is often required.
- Massaging and molding of the filler into place is at least as important as where the product is injected. Tell patients to avoid massaging on their own at home, which may displace the filler.
- Filler in the perioral region often benefits from injection to multiple regions. Lip filler helps soften vertical lip rhytids, and filling near the commissures can reduce the appearance of marionette lines.

Further reading

Niamtu J. Cosmetic Facial Surgery. 3rd edition. Elsevier; 2023.
Sclafani AP. Soft tissue fillers for management of the aging Perioral Complex. Facial Plast Surg 2005;21(01):74–8.
Ghavami A, Graivier M. Soft tissue fillers. In: Janis JJ, editor. Essentials of Aesthetic Surgery. New York: Thieme; 2018. p. 280–96.
Ali MJ, Ende K, Maas CS. Perioral rejuvenation and lip augmentation. Facial Plast Surg North Am 2007;15(4):491–500.
Kontis TC, Lacombe VG. Cosmetic injection techniques: a text and Video Guide to neurotoxins and fillers. New York: Thieme; 2019.
Sarnoff DS, Saini R, Gotkin RH. Comparison of filling agents for lip augmentation. Aesthet Surg J 2008;28(5):556–63.
Lupo MP, Smith SR, Thomas JA. Effectiveness of Juvéderm Ultra Plus dermal filler in the treatment of severe nasolabial folds. Plast Reconstr Surg 2008;121(1):289–97.
Perkins SW. The corner of the mouth lift and management of the oral commissure grooves. Facial Plast Surg Clin North Am 2007;15(4):471–6.

Disclosure

The authors have nothing to disclose.

Liquid Facelift

Maya D. Sinha, BS [a,1], Pradeep K. Sinha, MD, PhD [b,*]

KEYWORDS

- Liquid facelift • Non-surgical rejuvenation • Dermal fillers • Botulinum toxin • Botox • Hyaluronic acid • Minimally invasive
- Facial contouring

KEY POINTS

- The procedure involves the strategic placement of injectable fillers into specific areas to restore lost volume, lift sagging tissue, and smooth wrinkles.
- Concurrently, neurotoxins are used to relax dynamic muscles that contribute to expression lines, thereby enhancing the overall youthful appearance.
- May not be suitable for individuals with severe sagging or those seeking dramatic changes or surgically precise results.
- The outcomes are also temporary, requiring periodic maintenance treatments to sustain the effects.
- Incorrect placement or excessive use of fillers can result in complications such as infection, asymmetry, or the "overfilled" look.

Introduction

A liquid facelift is a non-surgical cosmetic procedure that uses injectable fillers and/or neurotoxin injection to refresh the face's appearance. Unlike a surgical facelift performed in an operating room under various forms of anesthesia, a liquid facelift is performed in an office chair, is less invasive, and offers quicker recovery times. The process involves injecting a combination of dermal fillers such as hyaluronic acid and botulinum toxin to relax furrows caused by muscles of facial expression, smooth wrinkles in the facial skin, lift sagging areas, and restore lost volume. Newer fillers are approved to also enhance changes in bony contour and definition. The combined effects can last from 6 months to 2 years, depending on the filler type and individual's metabolism. However, a liquid facelift is nonetheless temporary and requires ongoing maintenance. It is an ideal choice for those seeking a youthful look without the risks and downtime associated with surgery.

The whole process typically takes less than 30 minutes, depending on the extent of the treatment. The results can be seen almost immediately, with final results typically visible within 2 weeks once any swelling has subsided and the neurotoxins have reached full effect.

Neurotoxins

The currently available neurotoxin products in the United States include

1. OnabotulinumtoxinA (Botox Cosmetic®): The most well-known brand and is used for a variety of cosmetic and medical conditions, such as wrinkles, excessive sweating, and chronic migraines.
2. AbobotulinumtoxinA (Dysport®): Similar to OnabotulinumA and is used for wrinkles and muscle spasticity.
3. IncobotulinumtoxinA (Xeomin®): Used for wrinkles, blepharospasm, cervical dystonia, and other conditions.
4. PrabotulinumtoxinA (Jeuveau®): A newer addition to the group and is specifically approved for the temporary improvement in the appearance of moderate to severe frown lines.
5. RimabotulinumtoxinB (Myobloc®): Primarily used for the treatment of cervical dystonia and chronic sialorrhea and is not typically used for cosmetic procedures. Does not require refrigeration for storage.
6. DaxibotulinumA (Daxxify): A newer peptide-enhanced neuromodulator which can last 6 to 9 months with a single treatment session.

Neurotoxin injections, such as Botox Cosmetic®, are commonly used in cosmetic procedures to reduce wrinkles and fine lines. While they are generally safe, they can cause side effects, including bruising, swelling, headaches, drooping eyelids or eyebrows, flu-like symptom, dry eyes, or excessive tearing or allergic reactions. Though rare, some people may have an allergic reaction to the neurotoxin, resulting in rash, itching, or shortness of breath.[1-4] In rare cases, the effects of the neurotoxin may spread beyond the treatment area, causing more serious symptoms such as muscle weakness, vision problems, and difficulty speaking or swallowing, When the brain sends a signal for a muscle to contract, it is sent via the nervous system and neurotransmitters, primarily acetylcholine, carry this signal across the synapses to the muscle fibers. When acetylcholine attaches to receptors on the muscle cells, it causes the cells to contract, or shorten, resulting in a muscle movement. When a neurotoxin is injected, it binds to high affinity receptors and enters the cell where it is cleaved. The

[a] Emory University School of Medicine, 100 Woodruff Circle, Atlanta, GA 30322, USA
[b] Private Practice, Atlanta, GA, USA
* Corresponding author.
E-mail address: drsinha@drsinha.com
[1] Present address: 5730 Glenridge Drive, Suite T200, Atlanta, GA 30328.

light chain interacts with synaptosomal-associated protein (SNAP 24) and syntaxin where it prevents the fusion of acetylcholine vesicles with the cell membrane and thus release of acetylcholine at the neuromuscular junction, thereby stopping the signal transmission from the nerve to the muscle.[5] With the signal blocked, the muscle can no longer contract. This leads to a temporary reduction in muscle activity, which can smooth wrinkles and prevent the formation of new ones. Given the number of mimetic muscles of the face (Fig. 1), there are several options to soften or eliminate wrinkles caused by repetitive movement or excess tone. As well, understanding of how muscles work in pairs allows additional options for facial rejuvenation. For example, the brow is elevated by the frontalis muscle and depressed by the lateral portion of the orbicularis oculi, procerus, and corrugator supercilii muscles. By relaxing these brow depressor muscles with botulinum toxin injections, the brow can be elevated by "untethering" the frontalis muscle. Similar elevation of the angle of the mouth can be achieved by releasing the zygomaticus major and minor muscles from the counter action of the depressor anguli oris muscle. Drawing from injection patterns used for treating hemifacial spasm and facial paralysis, selectively relaxing muscles that "releases" other mimetic muscles can help achieve another level of facial rejuvenation. Conversely, there is also the concept of "recruitment" where, after injection of botulinum toxin, adjacent muscles increase in tone and may require additional injections for best aesthetic effect, for example, increase in "bunny lines" on the nose after injection of the glabella area.

In the context of a liquid facelift, generally, neurotoxins are used in the upper one-third of the face to diminish wrinkles associated with expressive facial muscle movement, however, benefits across the entire face and neck can be achieved for advanced injectors (Fig. 2). The most common areas include the lines caused by the corrugator and procerus muscles in the glabella (the "11's"), horizontal forehead lines caused by the frontalis muscle, and lateral radiating lines from the eyes caused by the orbicularis oculi muscle.

Additionally, rejuvenating effects of neurotoxins in other areas of the face can further enhance appearance. These areas include eliminating "bunny lines" in the nose, dimpled chin ("peau d'orange"), and neck bands from the platysma muscle. Some youthful enhancements can be achieved with the mouth by improving upper lip pout via injections in the orbicularis oris muscle ("lip flip") and decreasing excessive gingival show ("gummy smile") via injections in levator labii superioris alaeque nasi muscles. A summary of common injection sites is shown in Fig. 2.

Neurotoxins can be injected in the masseter and temporalis muscles to decrease muscle tightness and spasm from temporomandibular joint (TMJ) syndrome. Repetitive injections to maintain relief from TMJ syndrome (Fig. 3) has resulted in a noticeable decrease in muscle mass and, in concert with midface dermal fillers, result in conversation of a "pear" appearance of the face (flat cheeks and prominent masseter muscles) to restoration of the "apple" shape of the face with prominent cheeks and tapering jaw on anterior view.

Dermal Fillers

Absence of wrinkles and the presence of convexities that infer plumpness and light reflection are an important component of youthful appearance. These features are due in part to fullness of fat pads in the face (Fig. 4). Loss of soft tissue (Fig. 5) and bony volume (Fig. 6) is intrinsic to the facial aging process and creates wrinkles and convexities. Injectable fillers provide an opportunity to correct volume loss in these areas. The Food and Drug Administration (FDA) had approved several types of dermal fillers for use in facial cosmetic procedures. These include.

1. Hyaluronic Acid Fillers: This category includes product families such Juvederm®, Restylane®, Belotero®, and Revanesse® Versa. Hyaluronic acid is a naturally occurring substance in the body that helps add volume and hydration to the skin. These fillers are often used for smoothing and contouring facial wrinkles and folds, lip augmentation, and reducing under-eye shadows.[6]
2. Calcium Hydroxylapatite Fillers: Radiesse® is a prominent filler in this category, often used for smoothing moderate to severe creases such as nasolabial folds, marionette lines, and for enhancing fullness of the cheeks.[7]
3. Poly-L-lactic Acid Fillers: Sculptra Aesthetic® falls under this category. It is a biodegradable, biocompatible synthetic material used to replace lost collagen, generally used in the lower face for deep facial wrinkles and folds.
4. Polymethylmethacrylate (PMMA) Fillers: Bellafill® is one of these fillers. It is used to treat medium-to-deep wrinkles, folds, and furrows, particularly nasolabial folds. It can also

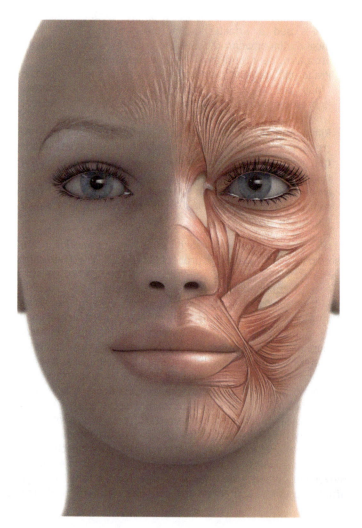

Fig. 1 Mimetic muscles of the face. (*From* iStock.com/t.light.)

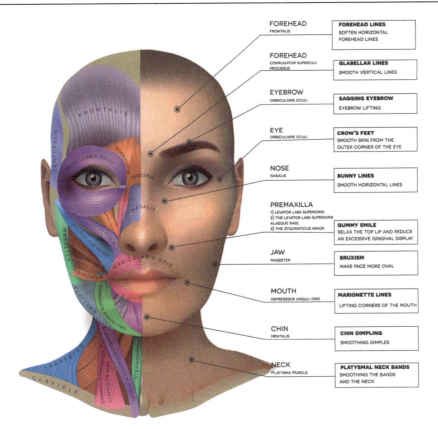

Fig. 2 Common uses for botulinum toxin in the face with associated target muscles. (*From* iStock.com/TefiM.)

be used for lip augmentation and to diminish the appearance of acne scars.
5. Autologous Fat Injections: These are not brand-name fillers but rather a procedure where fat is taken from one area of the patient's body and then injected into areas of the face to restore volume.

The Juvéderm® collection of dermal fillers is designed to meet each patient's aesthetic goals and the products can be differentiated based on technology. Hylacross is the original homogenized manufacturing technology, FDA approved in 2006, and includes Juvéderm® Ultra and Juvéderm® Ultra Plus. Hylacross technology utilizes a high concentration of cross-linked hyaluronic acid (HA) molecules with identical molecular weights.[8] Ultra is used for lips while Ultra Plus is used for fine lines.[8–10] The newest Vycross technology, FDA approved in 2013, utilizes a mixture of high and low molecular weight HA molecules with enhanced cross-linking to create a smoother filler accompanied by reduced pain and swelling among patients after treatment. This new technology is designed to restore volume loss, smooth fine lines and wrinkles, and restore contours.[11] The Vycross dermal fillers include Voluma, Volbella, Volux, and Vollure. Voluma is used for the cheeks and chin.[6] Volbella for the undereye and lips.[6,9,10] Volux for the jawline,[12] and Vollure for fine lines and wrinkles.[9,10]

Another well-known collection of dermal fillers is Restylane®. Each product is composed of hyaluronic acid derived from bacterial fermentation and are crosslinked with 1,4-butanediol diglycidylether (BDDE),[13,14] but they vary in their degree of crosslinking, gel particle size, and indicated use.[15] The Restylane portfolio is based on 2 technologies: non-animal stabilized hyaluronic acid (NASHA) and XpresHAn Technology. XpresHAn Technology is also known as Optimal Balance Technology (OBT) outside of the United States. These 2 technologies create a more versatile range of treatments that allows providers to individualize results.[16] The NASHA gels are firmer, create definition, have a distinct lifting capacity, and are most suitable for defining the jawline, lifting cheeks, and reducing wrinkles.[13,16,17] XpresHAn Technology is characterized by flexibility and distributed product integration. Dermal fillers that use this technology can adapt to dynamic facial expressions and are ideal for lips, cheek wrinkles, nasolabial folds, and marionette lines.[16–18] Traditional Restylane®, Restylane®-L, Restylane® Defyne, Restylane®

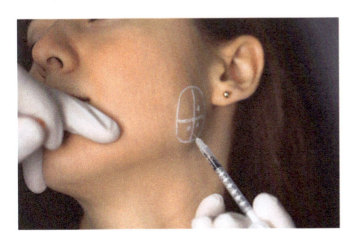

Fig. 3 Target area for masseter muscle injections for temporomandibular joint (TMJ) relief and to soften muscle bulge. (*From* iStock.com/Emir Hoyman.)

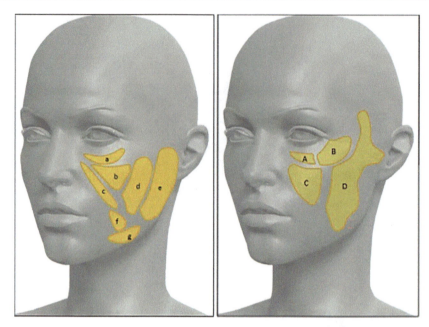

Fig. 4 Superficial cheek fat compartments: (a) Infraorbital fat. (b) Medial cheek fat. (c) Nasolabial fat. (d) Middle cheek fat. (e) Lateral cheek fat. (f) Superior jowl fat. (g) Inferior jowl fat. Deep cheek fat compartments: (*A*) Medial sub-orbicularis oculi fat. (*B*) Lateral sub-orbicularis oculi fat. (*C*) Deep medial cheek fat. (*D*) Buccal fat. (*From* Fundarò S (2018) Anatomy and aging of cheek fat compartments, Med Dent Res. 2: https://doi.org/10.15761/MDR.1000111.

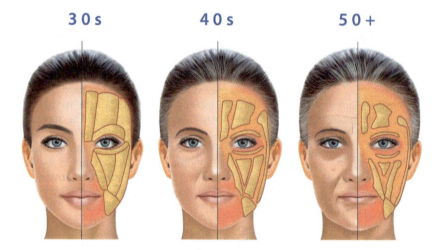

Fig. 5 "Deflation" of facial fats pads during the aging process. (Allergan, ND-JUV-2050028, Feb 2020. With permission from AbbVie.)

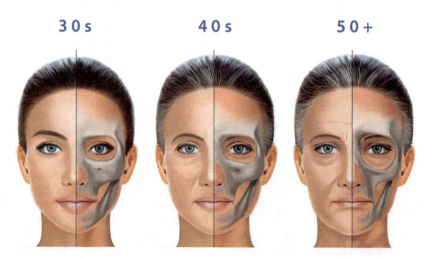

Fig. 6 Bony mass volume reduction during the aging process. (Allergan, ND-JUV-2050028, Feb 2020. With permission from AbbVie.)

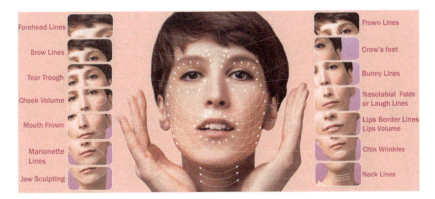

Fig. 7 Common applications for dermal fillers. (*From* iStock.com/Marina113.)

Lyft with lidocaine, and Restylane® Refyne are indicated for correction of moderate to severe facial wrinkles and folds, for example, nasolabial folds. Restylane® Lyft with lidocaine is also indicated for cheek augmentation, restoration of midface contour deficiencies, and correction of volume deficits in the dorsal hand.[17,18] Restylane® Contour is indicated for cheek augmentation and correction of midface contour deficiencies. Restylane® Kysse and Restylane® Silk are indicated for injection into the lips for lip augmentation and correction of the upper perioral rhytids.[17] Restylane® Eyelight can improve infraorbital hollowing.[19]

Knowledge regarding the etiology of facial aging changes has evolved from a gravitational theory to an increasing understanding that aging is complex, dynamic, multifactorial, and an integrated process.[20,21] The discovery that facial fat pads exist as many dynamic compartments, as opposed to 1 homogenous mass represents a breakthrough in the understanding of facial aging. In 2000, Donofrio brought attention to the "compartmentalized" appearance of the clinically aging face. She proposed that periorbital, buccal, and perioral fat tend to atrophy, while submental, jowl, nasolabial, and lateral malar regions tend to hypertrophy.[22] In 2007, Lambros illustrated the fundamental role of volume loss and deflation in the aged face through a longitudinal photographic analysis of 130 patients over an average period of 25 years.[23] In the same year, Rohrich and Pessa elucidated facial fat compartmentalization.[24] Since then, many subsequent studies have built upon this body of knowledge. These studies are summarized in a textbook published by Pessa and Rohrich.[25] These facial compartments can be evaluated and augmented to achieve restoration of natural volume distribution.[26]

An aging face undergoes a spectrum of changes, which may present as sunken or may predominate as tissue droop or fat bulges. Over time, the facial fat compartments in the upper and middle thirds of the face tend to thin with age, or atrophy.[20,22] In the forehead and glabellar area, the predominant signs of aging include wrinkle formation and an increase in nasofrontal angle that flattens and decreases projection.[27,28] Other signs of aging in the upper two-thirds of the face include drooping eyebrow and eyelids, infraorbital hollowing, globe retrusion, crow's feet, and deepening of nasolabial folds. Wrinkle formation may be compounded by fat loss. The lower third of the face tends to become progressively thicker, or hypertrophy.[20,22] As deeper fat pads decrease with age, this reduces their support of more superficial fat pads, which can then begin to sag, contributing to the development of perioral lines and folds. Prominent signs of aging in the bottom thirds of the face include "marionette" lines, loss of definition in the jawline, and jowl formation.[20] The fat pads also become more distinguishable, rather than blending naturally with the overall shape of your face (see Fig. 5). While it is impossible to stop this natural process, a good skincare regime can improve overall elasticity and firmness, to counteract the effects of fat pad changes. As always, good sun protection, staying hydrated, and not smoking[29] will also reduce the effects of aging.

Bony resorption and volume loss also figure significantly in the aging face (see Fig. 6). Deeper placement of appropriately thick fillers with good lifting capacity to restore bony prominences and anatomy is also the key to effectively utilizing fillers to address the aging face.

An effective option to replace the lost volume is to use dermal fillers to lift the areas of fat loss and restore volume. The aim of this treatment is to re-balance the fullness across your face. Thanks to detailed mapping of the superficial and deep facial fat pads, carried out in the late 2000s and early 2010s,[25] dermal fillers can now be used incredibly precisely and effectively to restore fullness in specific areas of volume loss (Fig. 7).

They can also restore the deeper fat pads, which, in turn, enables them to provide more support to the superficial fat pads and therefore both increase volume and reduce sagging. By targeting the underlying cause of volume loss and tailoring this approach to each patient's specific facial topography, it provides a far more natural result than simply using fillers to mask wrinkles.[26]

Plumping and refinement of lip anatomy further enhances facial appearance with the price use of fillers to augment and

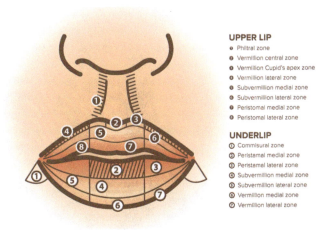

Fig. 8 Zones of the lip for filler injections. (*From* iStock.com/Greenni.)

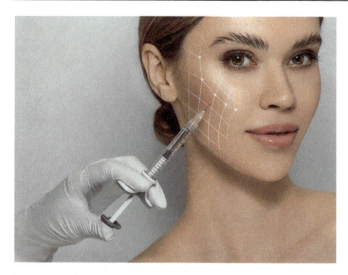

Fig. 9 Multiple microinjections of hyaluronic acid into cheek area, approximately 20 per side. (*From* iStock.com/peakSTOCK.)

highlight lip anatomy (Fig. 8). A newer use of hyaluronic acid injections involves using microdroplet injections to rejuvenate skin. One example is using Juvderm SkinVive (Volite). This pattern is usually performed in the cheek areas (Fig. 9).

Cautions

A thorough knowledge of muscle actions and vasculature of the face (Fig. 10) is imperative for safe injections. For botulinum toxin injections, it is possible to create untoward results when the injection infiltrates undesired muscles such as glabellar or brow injections causing inadvertent weakening of the muscles of the upper eyelid creating lid ptosis. This may be addressed with topical alpha-adrenergic eye drops and will usually subside in 2 to 4 weeks.

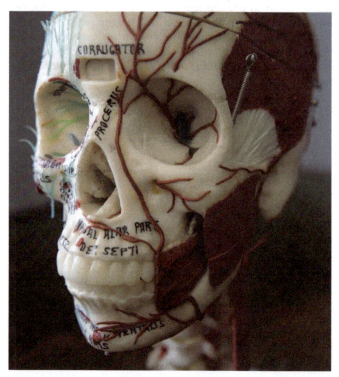

Fig. 10 Vessels prone to vascular compromise during filler injections. (*From* iStock.com/annedehaas.)

Failure to recognize pre-existing brow ptosis, for which the patient compensates with excessive frontalis muscle tone creating horizontal forehead lines, can lead to problems. Attempting to eliminate these lines with injections to the forehead will only unmask and exacerbate the ptosis leading to untoward brow drooping. This may be mitigated to some degree with the "Botox browlift" pattern described previously but will likely take 3 to 4 months to fully resolve.

More devastating complications can occur with filler injection. Direct intravascular injection or external compression of a vessel by extrinsic force from filler may lead to vascular compromise. This may result in ischemia of the skin supplied by the vessel. Often, patient complaints of bruising in the area are mistakenly dismissed as a normal aftermath of injections that will resolve quickly. Progressive discoloration, pain, and involvement of area adjacent to injection sites should clue the injector that something may be wrong. Rapid dissolution of filler with hyaluronidase, massage, and other use of anticoagulation as well as immediate referral to a surgical specialist are warranted. Emergent medications such as hyaluronidase, nitroglycerin paste, and aspirin must be kept handy and given based on medical history in case this is suspected.

Embolization of filler material when injecting the nasolabial fold or glabellar area may lead to central retinal vessel occlusion and blindness. Retro-ocular injection of hyaluronidase via a cannula or long needle and emergent ophthalmologic referral are important steps in decreasing the risk of permanent blindness.

Summary

Liquid facelift is a highly effective combination of neurotoxin and dermal filler injections that restore, refine, and rejuvenate the aging face in a cost-effective manner in the office. Duration of action and need for repetitive treatments to maintain results are important factors for patients to consider when comparing these procedures to other modalities such as cosmetic laser treatments and surgery. Liquid facelift gives medical practitioners another highly effective and popular tool to address the aging face when designed and performed correctly.

Clinics care points

- Office-based injections can address several aging face processes including wrinkles caused by mimetic muscles, soft tissue volume loss, and bony volume loss.
- A thorough understanding of facial anatomy, including muscles, fat pads, and bony prominences, is key to achieving excellent, natural looking results.
- Vascular compromise, excessive weaking of target, or adjacent mimetic muscles or asymmetric volumizing can lead to poor or devastating results.
- Liquid Facelift techniques are powerful tools in facial rejuvenation but have limitations as compared to other techniques including surgery, lasers, or other aesthetic devices. Proper counseling of all available options for patients is essential for achieving the best outcomes for patients.

Acknowledgments

The authors would like to acknowledge and thank Sierra Hyland for her valuable assistance with the article.

Disclosure

The authors have nothing to disclose.

References

1. Silverstein P. Smoking and wound healing. Am J Med 1992;93(1):S1.
2. Lafaille P, Benedetto A. Fillers: Contraindications, side effects and Precautions. J Cutan Aesthet Surg 2010;3(1):16–9.
3. Bitterman-Deutsch O, Kogan L, Nasser F. Delayed immune mediated adverse effects to hyaluronic acid fillers: report of five cases and review of the literature. Dermatol Report 2015;7:5851.
4. U.S. Food and Drug Administration. (n.d.). Dermal Filler DO's and Don'ts for Wrinkles, Lips and More. https://www.fda.gov/consumers/consumer-updates/dermal-filler-dos-and-donts-wrinkles-lips-and-more#:~:text=Most%20side%20effects%20associated%20with,Bruising.
5. Sellin LC. The pharmacological mechanism of botulism. Trends Pharmacol Sci 1985;6:80–2.
6. Goodman GJ, Swift A, Remington BK. Current concepts in the Use of Voluma, Volift, and Volbella. Plast Reconstr Surg 2015;136:139S.
7. Trinh LN, Gupta A. Non-hyaluronic acid fillers for midface augmentation: a Systematic review. Facial Plast Surg 2021;37(4):536–42.
8. Bogdan Allemann I, Baumann L. Hyaluronic acid gel (Juvéderm) preparations in the treatment of facial wrinkles and folds. Clin Interv Aging 2008;3(4):629–34.
9. Pierre S, Liew S, Bernardin A. Basics of dermal filler rheology. Dermatol Surg 2015;41(Suppl 1):S120–6.
10. Hee CK, Shumate GT, Narurkar V, et al. Rheological properties and in Vivo performance characteristics of soft tissue fillers. Dermatol Surg 2015;41(Suppl 1):S373–81.
11. Calvisi L, Gilbert E, Tonini D. Rejuvenation of the perioral and lip regions with two new dermal fillers: the Italian experience with Vycross™ Technology. J Cosmet Laser Ther 2017;19(1):54–8.
12. Bertossi D, Robiony M, Lazzarotto A, et al. Nonsurgical Redefinition of the chin and jawline of Younger Adults with a hyaluronic acid filler: results evaluated with a Grid system approach. Aesthet Surg J 2021;41(9):1068–76.
13. Kablik J, Monheit GD, Yu L, et al. Comparative physical properties of hyaluronic acid dermal fillers. Dermatol Surg 2009;35:302–12.
14. Molliard GS, Albert S, Mondon K. Key importance of compression properties in the biophysical characteristics of hyaluronic acid soft-tissue fillers. J Mech Behav Biomed Mater 2016;61:290–8. Restylane, https://www.restylaneusa.com/.
15. Segura S, Anthonioz L, Fuchez F, et al. A complete range of hyaluronic acid filler with distinctive physical properties specifically designed for optimal tissue adaptations. J Drugs Dermatol 2012;11(1 Suppl):s5–8.
16. Refine the science behind Restylane. Science behind restylane. 2021. Accessed August 13, 2023.
17. Di Gregorio C, Gauglitz G, Partridge J. Individualized treatment Algorithm using hyaluronic acid fillers for lifting, contouring and volumizing the midface. Clin Cosmet Investig Dermatol 2022 Apr 14;15:681–90.
18. Solish N, Bertucci V, Percec I, et al. Dynamics of hyaluronic acid fillers formulated to maintain natural facial expression. J Cosmet Dermatol 2019;18:738–46.
19. Restylane Healthcare Professionals. Instructions for Use Restylane Eyelight. 2023. Accessed August 13, 2023.
20. Swift A, Liew S, Weinkle S, et al. The facial aging process from the "inside out". Aesthet Surg J 2021;41(10):1107–19.
21. Wan D, Amirlak B, Rohrich R, et al. The clinical importance of the fat compartments in midfacial aging. Plast Reconstr Surg Glob Open 2014;1(9):e92.
22. Donofrio LM. Fat distribution: a morphologic study of the aging face. Dermatol Surg 2000;26:1107–12.
23. Lambros V. Observations on periorbital and midfacial aging. Plast Reconstr Surg 2007;120:1367–76.
24. Rohrich RJ, Pessa JE. The fat compartments of the face: anatomy and clinical implications for cosmetic surgery. Plast Reconstr Surg 2007;119:2219–27.
25. Pessa JE, Rohrich RJ. Facial topography. Clinical anatomy of the face. St Louis (MO): Quality Medical Publishing, Inc; 2012.
26. Fitzgerald R, Rubin AG. Filler placement and the fat compartments. Dermatol Clin 2014;32(1):37–50.
27. Rossi AM, Eviatar J, Green JB, et al. Signs of facial aging in men in a diverse, multinational study: timing and preventive behaviors. Dermatol Surg 2017;43(Suppl 2):S210–20.
28. Alexis AF, Grimes P, Boyd C, et al. Racial and ethnic differences in self-assessed facial aging in women: results from a multinational study. Dermatol Surg 2019;45(12):1635–48.
29. Yazdanparast T, Hassanzadeh H, Nasrollahi SA, et al. Cigarettes smoking and skin: a comparison study of the biophysical properties of skin in smokers and non-smokers. Tanaffos 2019 Feb;18(2):163–8.

Nonsurgical Rhinoplasty with Hyaluronic Acid

Cang Carson Huynh, MD, DMD*, Christopher Hamamdjian, DO

KEYWORDS

- Nose filler • Nonsurgical rhinoplasty • Nonsurgical nose job • Nose injection • Nose augmentation • Liquid rhinoplasty

KEY POINTS

- Minor nose contour deficiency and irregularities can be corrected with injection of hyaluronic acid fillers as an alternative to surgical rhinoplasty
- Nonsurgical rhinoplasty is a safe and affordable treatment with little to no down time
- Nonsurgical rhinoplasty treatment has a high patient satisfaction rate with careful patient selection and management of expectations.
- Precautions should be taken to avoid overinjection of filler for nose augmentation. There is a small margin of error for natural looking esthetic results.

Introduction: Nature of the Problem

The history of nonsurgical rhinoplasty with hyaluronic acid fillers dates back to the early 2000s when medical advancements in cosmetic dermatology began exploring less-invasive alternatives to traditional surgical procedures. Hyaluronic acid, a naturally occurring substance in the body known for its hydrating and volumizing properties, was already being used successfully in other facial augmentation treatments. This prompted researchers and practitioners to experiment with its application in reshaping and enhancing the nose without resorting to surgery.

During the mid-2000s, the use of hyaluronic acid fillers for nonsurgical rhinoplasty gained momentum. This approach offered several advantages, including minimal downtime, reduced risks, and temporary results that allowed for adjustments over time. By injecting hyaluronic acid fillers into precise areas of the nose, cosmetic practitioners could effectively smooth out irregularities, correct minor asymmetry, and augment the nasal bridge, and enhancing tip projection and definition. Over the years, refinements in technique and an increasing understanding of facial anatomy have led to improved outcomes, making nonsurgical rhinoplasty with hyaluronic acid fillers a popular choice for those seeking subtle nasal enhancements without the commitment of surgery.

Patient selection:
Dorsal augmentation for low dorsum to increase dorsal height and contour
Round tip with low projection
Radix deficiency
Minor contour irregularity from prior rhinoplasty
Iatrogenic over resection of dorsal hump

Radiance Surgery & Aesthetic Medicine, 6133 Peachtree Dunwoody Road, Atlanta, GA 30328, USA
* Corresponding author.
E-mail address: atlantafacemd@gmail.com

Relative contraindications:
Nonrealistic expectations
Excessively thin skin
Preexisting nasal implant

Technique

Material list: HA fillers, Hylenex, disinfectant, topical anesthetic cream (LMX4 or lidocaine-prilocaine), BD syringe, 27G needle, gauze, Arnicare (Newtown Square, PA), cotton applicator, chlorhexadine, vibration wand, and camera (Fig. 1).

Evaluation and assessment should be done to predetermine the amount of filler needed for a particular patient. Most patients with minor contour irregularity requires less than 1 mL of filler. Use 1-mL sterile BD syringe to transfer product if using 0.5 mL or less with 27G needle included with packaging.

Take pretreatment photos.
Clean skin with alcohol prior to applying topical anesthetic for 10 minutes.
Second skin prep with chlorhexidine (Fig. 2).
Using nondominant hand, stabilize syringe as necessary to achieve desired injection angulation, and a vibration device can provide additional patient comfort (Fig. 3).

Injection of filler in radix and dorsum while tenting up skin with nondominant hand (Fig. 4). In Asian patients and those with more obtuse nasofrontal angles, use horizontal position of the supratarsal crease as a guide for upper limit of filler product placement and starting point of dorsal transition.

Slow and gentle injection of not more than 0.1 mL of product at each injection site along midline of nose is performed. Walk needle down caudally along dorsum with small aliquots of product to blend into lower dorsum. Inject only what is necessary to blend contour into the supratip contour. Any product placement into the lower dorsum and supratip

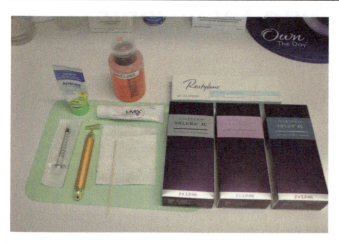

Fig. 1 Material list: HA fillers, Hylenex, disinfectant, topical anesthetic cream (LMX4 or lidocaine-prilocaine), BD syringe, 27G needle, gauze, Arnicare, cotton applicator, chlorhexadine, vibration wand.

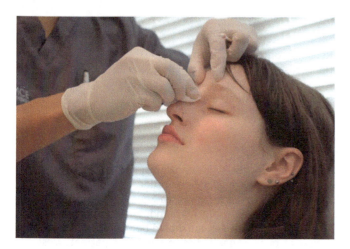

Fig. 2 Second skin prep with chlorhexadine.

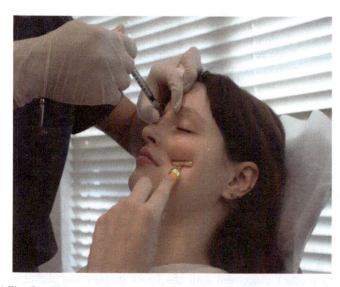

Fig. 3 Using nondominant hand stabilize syringe as necessary to achieve desired injection angulation and a vibration device can provide additional patient comfort.

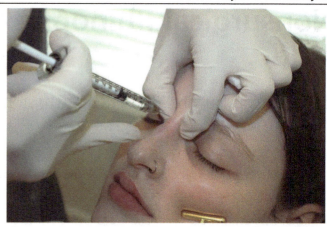

Fig. 4 Injection of filler in radix and dorsum while tenting up skin with nondominant hand.

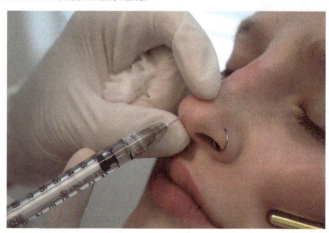

Fig. 5 During nasal tip injections, it is important to stay midline to minimize risk of intravascular injection or perivascular compression. Filler can be placed through the interdomal ligament and gentle injection as the needle is withdrawn to create a column of product supporting the tip.

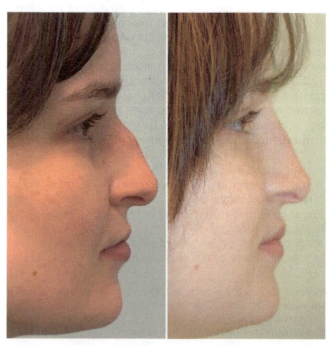

Fig. 6 Preprocedural/Postprocedural oblique and lateral photos depicting improved dorsal contouring, light reflection and tip definition.

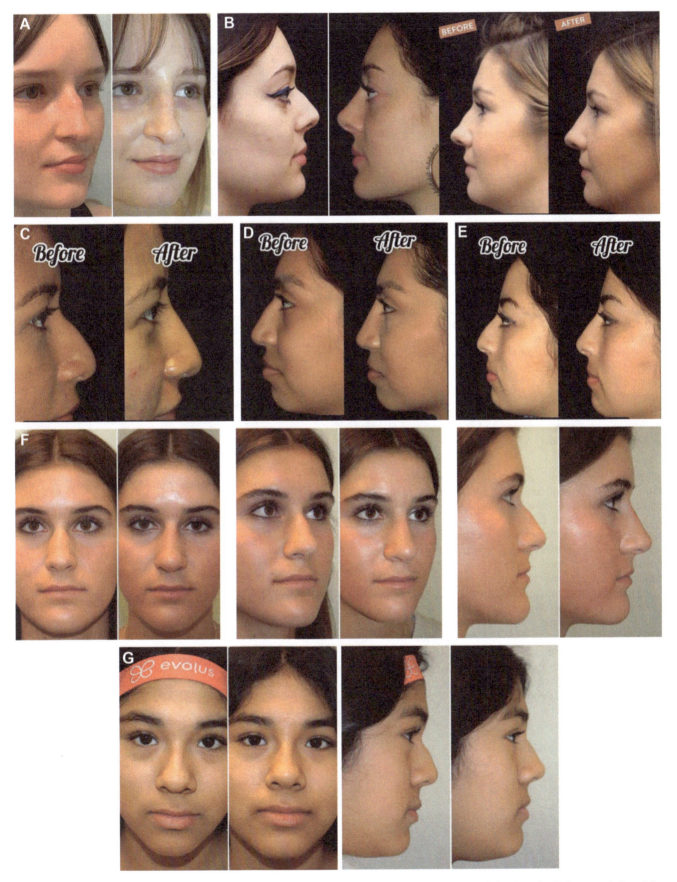

Fig. 7 Clinical results. (A) Prominent dorsal hump refined postprocedure with enhanced tip definition (B–E) Improved dorsal hump contouring, (F) enhanced nasal dorsal esthetic lines, light reflection, dorsal hump reduction, and nasal tip definition as visualized from frontal, oblique, and lateral views, and (G) teenage patient with improved nasal light reflection and enhanced contouring to dorsal hump. Fig. 7 [B, C, D, E]: *Courtesy* of Dr Cang, Carson Huynh MD, DMD, FACS, FAACS.

area can create a lowering effect on the relative tip projection.

When injection the tip, it is also important to stay midline to minimize the risk of intravascular injection or perivascular compression. Filler can be placed through the interdomal ligament and gently injected as the needle is withdrawn to create a column of product supporting the tip (Fig. 5). Typically, not more than 0.1 mL of product is needed here. Additional 0.1 to 0.2 mL of product may be placed directly on the domal cartilages at the midline to gain additional tip projection.

Patients with large pores will have a limited volume of product that is able to be placed in the tip area because the injection pressure of excess product will extrude through the pores.

- Hold gentle pressure with cotton gauze for minor bleeding points as needed.
- Apply Arnica gel and roll out any contour irregularities with cotton applicator. The gel also helps to occlude minor bleeding points on the skin.
- Assess patient from multiple angles to ensure symmetry and satisfactory contour. Ask the patient to look in the mirror to gain input and approval of contours.
- Take immediate posttreatment photos.
- Review posttreatment instructions:
  - Gentle face washing taking care not to apply excessive pressure over treated areas.
  - Eyeglasses may be worn as long as nosepieces are resting laterally on the nasal bones and not directly contacting the midline dorsum.

Follow-up revaluation for patient's satisfaction with 2 weeks to look for any contour irregularities or asymmetry issues to be addressed. It is not uncommon for patients to request additional product for augmentation even though they are satisfied with the result. It is especially important to manage the patient's expectation at this time by reviewing previous discussion of limitation of filler being a soft gel in nose augmentation. A common pitfall to avoid is overinjection resulting in local displacement of filler cephalically or laterally, resulting in unnatural nasofrontal contour and excessive width of the dorsal esthetic lines.

Patients with higher expectations for more dramatic results can be recommended for surgical augmentation rhinoplasty with autogenous grafts or dorsal implants.

Results should be reevaluated after 6 months to determine whether touch up treatments are needed. Many patients are able to maintain satisfactory results beyond 1 year, some up to 2 years.

Surgical technique

Preoperative Planning

Evaluation and assessment should be done to predetermine the amount of filler needed for a particular patient. Preoperative photos should be taken for documentation and should include frontal, oblique, profile, and worm's eye views. The nose should be evaluated for general contour, symmetry, skin thickness, and distensibility. Photo simulation application such as Body Editor may be helpful in discussing expectation of treatment outcome with patients.

Prep and Patient Positioning

Nonsurgical nose augmentation has a high rate of acceptance and patient satisfaction due to affordability, quick procedure chair time, little to no down time, and relatively low risks. Potential complications can include excessive bleeding, bruising, intravascular injection leading to skin necrosis or ophthalmic complications. Other minor potential complications include contour asymmetry and irregularity, filler migration, or loss of augmentation effect resulting in patient dissatisfaction.

Pearls and Pitfalls

Careful patient selection and clear communication and management of the patient's expectations and keys to successful treatment outcome and satisfaction.

Use only nonpermanent hyaluronic acid fillers with high safety profile and dissolubility with hyaluronidase.

Stay midline and avoid injection in the highly vascular danger zones to minimize the risk of intravascular injections. It is better to err on undertreat rather than to overtreat during the initial treatment session. The margin for natural looking results is small, and it is easier to add more filler if needed at a follow-up visit than having to dissolve excess filler.

Underpromise and overdeliver. Those patients who want a larger amount of augmentation beyond the lifting limit of filler, or requesting significant changes to the tip should be recommended for surgical rhinoplasty.

Immediate postoperative care

Rehabilitation and Recovery

Apply anti-inflammatory topical gel (Arnicare) onto the treated area immediately and continue to use at home for next 24 to 48 hours.

Avoid facials or direct pressure to the nose during the first week. Patients can wear glasses or eyewear with nosepieces resting on lateral area of nose bridge. Avoid direct contact of eyewear with the area treated with filler.

Patients are given instructions on how to gently massage any area of contour irregularity with a cotton tip applicator as needed.

Patient is given a follow-up visit appointment in 1 to 2 weeks to reevaluate results.

Clinical results

Case examples of before and after results.
Figures 6 and 7.

Summary

Soft tissue filler injections have the ability to provide predictable and life-altering effects—in part, this has caused them to become increasingly used in an array of esthetic applications. These products have the ability to augment the face and the nose is certainly no exception. The evolution of available products and clinical skill with the increased demand for rhinoplasty has led to these products being increasingly used for a nonsurgical approach of nasal contouring. For patients who are looking to enhance their facial esthetics without the need for traditional surgical procedures, this application in undeniably appealing. Their effects have the ability to provide dramatic changes, such as addressing dorsal hump deformities or even more fine adjustments such as adjusting nasal tip rotation. These hyaluronic acid-based products offer an immediate result with little to no interruption in a patient's daily life. From a safety standpoint, they offer the additional benefit of reversibility with hyaluronidase if needed. Although the effects are temporary, this approach proves to be of value for a myriad of reasons including to those patients who are uncertain pursuing a permanent result, unable to tolerate post-surgical downtime, or even afford the high price point of a traditional surgical rhinoplasty.

Clinics care points

- Careful patient selection and managing patient's expectations are keys to success.
- Use only hyaluronic acid fillers with high safety profile and dissolubility.
- Keep filler injection close to midline to mitigate potential vasular complications.
- Avoid overinjection of filler to avoid associated unwanted side effect with filler migration.

Further reading

Plastic surgery Statistics report. American Society of Plastic Surgeons. 2023 Available at:https://www.plasticsurgery.org/documents/News/Statistics/2020/plastic-surgery-statistics-full-report-2020.pdf Accessed September 6, 2023

Mehta U, Fridirici Z. Advanced techniques in nonsurgical rhinoplasty. Facial Plast Surg Clin North Am 2019;27:355–65.

Rohrich RJ, Agrawal N, Avashia Y, et al. Safety in the use of fillers in nasal augmentation—the liquid rhinoplasty. Plast Reconstr Surg Glob Open 2020;8:e2820.

Raggio BS, Asaria J. Filler rhinoplasty.StatPearls. Island (FL): StatPearls PublishingTreasure; 2021.

Williams LC, Kidwai SM, Mehta K, et al. Nonsurgical rhinoplasty: a systematic review of technique, outcomes, and complications. Plast Reconstr Surg 2020;146:41–51.

Kurkjian T, Jonathan MD, Ahmad J, et al. Soft-tissue fillers in rhinoplasty. Plast Reconstr Surg 2014;133:121e–6e.

Redaelli A. Medical rhinoplasty with hyaluronic acid and botulinum toxin a: a very simple and quite effective technique. J Cosmet Dermatol 2008;7:210–20.

Johnson ON, Kontis TC. Nonsurgical rhinoplasty. Facial Plast Surg 2016;32:500–6.

Rohrich RJ, Novak M, Cason R, et al. Soft tissue filler for secondary nasal deformities. Plast Reconstr Surg 2023. https://doi.org/10.1097/PRS.0000000000010747.

Rohrich R, Alleyne B, Novak M, et al. Nonsurgical rhinoplasty. Clin Plast Surg 2022;49(1):191–5. Epub 2021 Oct 9. PMID: 34782136.

Wright JM, Halsey JN, Rottgers SA. Dorsal augmentation: a review of current graft options. Eplasty 2023. 23:e4.

Josipovic LN, Sattler S, Schenck TL, et al. Five-point liquid rhinoplasty: results from a retrospective analysis of a novel standardized technique and considerations on safety. J Cosmet Dermatol 2022;21(11):5614–20.

Saad N, Stallworth CL. Liquid rhinoplasty. Facial Plast Surg Clin North Am 2022;30(3):357–64.

Kassir R, Venkataram A, Malek A, et al. Non-surgical rhinoplasty: the ascending technique and a 14-year retrospective study of 2130 cases. Aesthetic Plast Surg 2021;45(3):1154–68.

Periorbital Rejuvenation

Phillip Hooper Barbee, MD, DDS, MS [1]

KEYWORDS

- Periorbital rejuvenation • Periorbital filler • Tear trough filler • Midface volume correction • Periorbital neurotoxin • Liquid brow lift

KEY POINTS

- Neurotoxins can be used to elevate the brows and improve periorbital rhytids.
- Dermal fillers can be used to camouflage tear trough deformity.
- Correcting midface volume deficiency has a strong impact on the appearance of the periorbital region.

Introduction: nature of the problem

The periorbital region is often an area of concern for the aging-face patient population. The eyes are the main focal point of the face and aging in the structures surrounding the eyes can be particularly concerning for many patients. As with any part of the body, an understanding of the underlying anatomic and physiologic aspects of aging is critical for determining the correct diagnosis and rendering the most appropriate treatment.

The highly dynamic muscles of facial expression surrounding the eyes predispose the periorbital skin to both static and dynamic rhytids. Additionally, the extremely thin skin of the eyelids is highly susceptible to dermatochalasis, or excess skin formation. Dermatochalasis can occur in the upper eyelids, lower eyelids, or both. In the upper eyelid, dermatochalasis can be accentuated when brow ptosis is also present. In the lower eyelid, dermatochalasis can be accentuated with pseudoherniation of the orbital fat pads.

Fat pseudoherniation occurs as the orbital septum begins to weaken and the orbital fat pads pseudoherniate from the bony orbit. It presents as heavy "eye bags" and a telltale sign of this condition is a patient who complains about looking tired even when they are well rested. Weakening of the orbital septum can occur prematurely in some younger patients who have a genetic predisposition to this condition. It occurs in both the upper and lower eyelids but is typically most noticeable in the lower eyelids.

The tear trough or nasojugal groove is a depression that forms at the junction of the lower eyelid and cheek. The appearance of this groove or depression is due to the attachments of the orbital retaining ligament which extends from the orbital rim to the dermis. The tear trough or nasojugal groove can become more apparent when both orbital pseudoherniation and midface volume loss are occurring simultaneously.

Upper eyelid rejuvenation

Rejuvenation of the upper eyelids with the use of injectables is achieved by modifying the position of the brow. Because brow ptosis increases crowding in the upper eyelid, the administration of neurotoxins to brow depressor muscles can achieve a lifting of the brow and stretching of the upper eyelid excess skin. The colloquially known "liquid brow lift" can be a powerful tool for patients with mild brow ptosis or dermatochalasis. An understanding of the brow-depressing and brow-elevating muscles is critical to achieving predictable lifting of the brows with neurotoxins.

The brow depressors are the orbicularis oculi, the corrugators supercili, and the procerus. The orbicularis oculi is the most powerful brow depressor. The only brow elevator is the frontalis muscle. The application of neurotoxins to the brow depressor muscles results in partial paralyzation of these muscles. When the brow-elevating frontalis muscle is left active, it is no longer countered by the depressor muscles with the result being elevation of the brow.

Lower eyelid rejuvenation

Rejuvenation of the lower eyelids with injectables can be achieved with neurotoxins and dermal fillers. Neurotoxins can be used to relax the orbicularis oculi which diminishes the appearance of periorbital rhytids. Specifically, lateral rhytids or "crow's feet." Some practitioners advocate the use of small doses of neurotoxins beneath the lower eyelid to halt the progression of crepey skin.

Dermal fillers are used in the rejuvenation of the lower eyelids to camouflage orbital fat pseudoherniation, tear trough deformity, and midface volume loss.

The orbital fat and midface fat can be thought of as "hills" whereas the tear trough can be thought of as a "valley." This notion of the "hill, valley, and hill" allows the practitioner to conceptualize where filler may be placed to smooth the transition between these components. Put simply, the addition of volume in the "valley" will not only diminish the appearance of the "valley" but also diminish the appearance of the "hill" on either side of the valley.

Surgical technique

Preoperative planning

A complete medical, surgical, and injectable history is the first step prior to any cosmetic procedure. Inquiring about a patient's

---

Facial Plastic & Reconstructive Surgery, 707 West Eau Gallie Boulevard, Melbourne, FL 32935, USA
E-mail address: drbarbee@drclevens.com
[1] 140 9th Avenue, Indialantic, FL, 32,903, USA.

past experience with injectables can give the provider an idea of the most appropriate treatment plan. Specifically, inquiry into the frequency and dosage of neurotoxin will allow the provider to prescribe the most appropriate plan for a given patient. A neurotoxin naive patient may be overwhelmed with a larger neurotoxin dose whereas an experienced patient may be dissatisfied by being underdosed.

It is recommended that a full set of photos including frontal, bilateral 3-quarter view, and bilateral lateral views are obtained (Figs. 1 and 2). The first step in treatment planning is to identify the patient's chief complaint. This can be accomplished by asking the patient to look in a hand mirror and point out what bothers them. For example, some patients may be bothered by brow ptosis and not by a tear trough deformity although both are present. Some patients may not be able to articulate exactly what it is that bothers them. In these cases, it is the provider's responsibility to accurately assess and educate the patient on their particular anatomy and physiology. Additionally, it is important to manage patient expectations. It should be made clear that injectable treatments typically do not yield the same level of results as surgical treatments. The patient should also be made aware that injectables are temporary and will require repeat treatments.

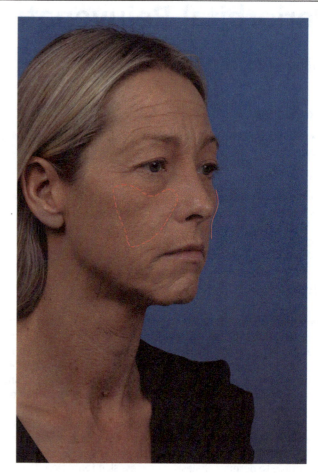

Fig. 2 Midface volume loss is best assessed on the 3-quarter view. The right side midface volume loss is outlined in by a red dashed line. The solid red line demonstrates the characteristic concave appearance of midface volume loss on the left side.

Surgical approach

For patients who will require both periorbital dermal filler and periorbital neurotoxin, it is advisable to place the filler prior to the neurotoxin. The dermal filler will often require some immediate manipulation and massage by the injector which can disrupt the precise placement of the neurotoxin. Ideally, there should be no manipulation of any region where neurotoxin has been administered to reduce the risk of migration.

Midface volume loss should be assessed and corrected prior to direct periorbital filler placement. Not only does correcting midface volume improve the overall aesthetics of the face, it often will indirectly improve the appearance of the under eye region.

Placing filler pre-periosteally, deep into the orbicularis muscle, and anterior to the inferior orbital rim yields the most predictable results while reducing the risk of adverse effects of the periorbital filler (edema, ecchymosis, contour irregularity, Tyndall effect). Placement of filler in this region can be accomplished with serial punctures and deposition of filler aliquots or retrograde linear threading. Linear threading can be accomplished with either a needle or a cannula. Some benefits of the cannula include less ecchymosis and less edema. The cannula also provides the injector with real-time visual and tactile feedback throughout the procedure. Needle deposition of filler aliquots should be reserved for patients with severe

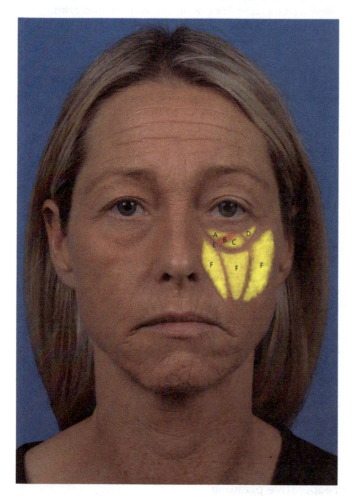

Fig. 1 The frontal view photograph demonstrates static rhytids, brow ptosis, upper and lower eyelid dermatochalasis, orbital fat pseudoherniation, tear trough deformity, and midface volume loss. (A) Nasal orbital fat pad. (B) Inferior oblique muscle. (C) Middle orbital fat pad. (D) Lateral orbital fat pad. (E) Tear trough. (F) Malar fat pads.

tear trough deformity and should serve as a foundation for linear threading.

Prep and patient positioning
Armamentarium
- 4 × 4 gauze
- Alcohol wipes
- 25-gauge needle
- 25-gauge cannula
- 27-gauge needle
- Marking pen or chalk pencil

Seat the patient in a 45° "beach chair" position
The periorbital region has a highly nuanced anatomy which can be altered by the effects of positioning and lighting. The patient should first be assessed in a neutral, upright position with ambient room lighting. Reclining the patient or applying bright lighting can obscure the subtleties of the regions where filler should most adequately be placed. However, it is difficult to perform procedures on patients in the upright seated position. To maintain an accurate presentation of the patient's anatomy and facilitate the ease of injection, a 45° seated position is advised. Ensuring that the patient's head is well supported with a headrest will provide stability to the regions being treated.

Place a 4 × 4 gauze and alcohol pad on the patient's shoulders
Having gauze and alcohol pads immediately adjacent to the injection sites increases the efficiency of the procedure. Quick access to the alcohol pads allows the injector to cleanse the injection sites without leaving the patient's side. Having gauze immediately available is advantageous should any bleeding occur.

Surgical procedure
Midface filler
- Step 1: Midface injection marking
  - Fig. 3: Midface injection marking
  - Drawing lines from the lateral canthus to oral commissure and from the ala to the tragus creates an intersection which can be used as a rough guide to the ideal malar height of contour. Placing filler in the superior and lateral corner of this intersection creates a natural and feminine rejuvenation of the midface.
- Step 2: Midface filler technique
  - Cleanse the region with an alcohol wipe.
  - Lift the midface with the nondominant hand in the superolateral vector. With a 27-gauge needle loaded onto the filler syringe, introduce the needle perpendicular to the surface of the skin. Gently sound the zygomatic bone with the tip of the needle, retract slightly, and inject 0.2 mL to 0.3 mL aliquots of filler in the supraperiosteal space. Reassess the periorbital region after midface volume correction to determine the volume of filler needed for correction.

Tear trough filler
- Step 1: Tear trough injection marking
  - Fig. 4: Tear trough injection marking
  - Mark the junction of the midpupillary line and a horizontal line extending from the nasal ala. This location

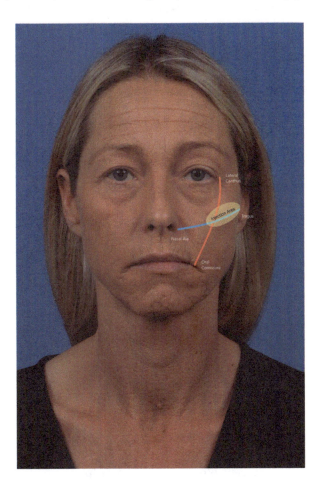

Fig. 3 Midface injection marking.

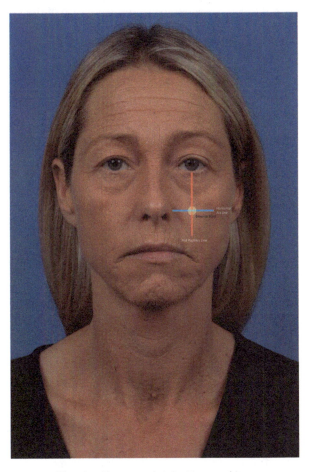

Fig. 4 Tear trough injection marking.

provides a reliable and repeatable access point for the placement of tear trough periorbital filler.
- Step 2: Pierce skin with a 25-gauge needle
  - Cleanse the region with an alcohol wipe.
  - The 25-gauge needle serves to create an access point for introducing the cannula through the skin.
  - The needle should enter perpendicular to the surface of the skin. Angling the needle upon entry to the skin can make it difficult for the cannula to enter the appropriate plane.
  - The needle should fully penetrate the dermis and barely enter the subcutaneous fat. Too superficial of a puncture will result in difficulty advancing the cannula whereas too deep of a puncture can result in unnecessary tissue trauma and bleeding.
  - Once the needle penetrates the dermis, it should be left in place. Introducing the needle and leaving it in place serves 2 purposes. First, it displaces the dermis providing an entry site for the cannula which will be maintained once the needle is removed. Second, it gives the assistant an opportunity to hand the injector the filler syringe and time to get into position for the injection.
- Step 3: Introduce the cannula
  - The injector should have their nondominant hand resting on the patient's cheek and the filler syringe in their dominant hand. Once the injector is ready, they will ask the assistant to slowly remove the 18-gauge needle. Allowing the assistant to remove the 18-gauge needle ensures that the injector will be in the ready position for introducing the cannula through the skin.
  - The cannula should enter perpendicular to the surface of the skin. It should follow the same path of the entry as the 18-gauge needle.
  - If the injector is experiencing difficulty entering the hole made by the 18-gauge needle, gently squeezing the region will create a small flash of blood which can aid in identifying the hole.
- Step 4: Superficial musculoaponeurotic system (SMAS) penetration
  - The cannula will continue to be advanced until slight resistance and a gentle release are felt. This represents penetration through the SMAS layer.
  - Once the cannula has penetrated the SMAS, the cannula will be angled superiorly and advanced into the region of the tear trough.
- Step 5: Retrograde linear threading
  - Fig. 5: Tear trough filler technique
  - Gentle lifting of the cannula and palpating it with the nondominant hand provides the injector with feedback as to the exact location of the cannula tip.
  - 0.1 mL linear threads placed in a retrograde fashion perpendicular to the course of the tear trough will serve as a scaffolding that elevates the orbicularis oculi muscle in the region of the tear trough.
- Step 6: Massage and reassessment
  - After several threads have been placed, the filler will likely require some massage to achieve a smooth appearance.
  - Once the filler has been manually smoothed, the injector will reassess the region for any voids or deficiencies that require additional filler.

Glabella and Periorbital Neurotoxin
- Step 1: Glabella and periorbital neurotoxin marking
  - Fig. 6: Glabella and periorbital neurotoxin

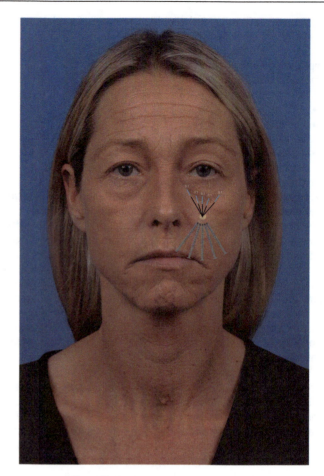

Fig. 5 Tear trough filler technique.

- Asking the patient to "make an angry face" will prompt them to activate the brow depressor muscles.
- While the patient is animating, mark the procerus and corrugator supercilii.
- Mark the orbicularis oculi just beneath the tail of the brow.
- Continue marking the orbicularis oculi circumferentially in the lateral and inferior regions of the muscle.
- Step 2
  - Inject 2 to 4 units of botulinum toxin type A into each site.
  - Figs. 7 and 8: 2 weeks post-treatment with hyaluronic acid (HA) filler (1 syringe per cheek, 1 syringe per periorbital region) and 44 units of botulinum toxin type A to the glabella and periorbital regions. Notice the improvement in midface volume and periorbital contour as well as elevation of brows.

Potential complications
Levator palpebrae superioris & muller's muscle ptosis
Avoiding ptosis when using botulinum toxin for cosmetic purposes, especially in the forehead and brow area, requires careful injection techniques and an understanding of the anatomy involved. Providers should avoid injecting too close to the eyebrow or the eyelid margin to reduce the risk of affecting the muscles that control eyelid elevation.

Frontalis-dependent ptosis
Frontalis-dependent ptosis, also known as "pseudo-ptosis" or "compensatory ptosis," occurs when the frontalis muscle

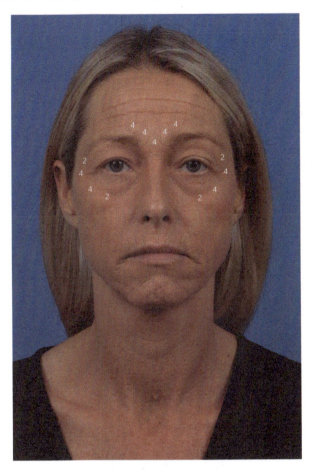

Fig. 6 Glabella and periorbital neurotoxin.

compensates for a ptotic upper eyelid or brow. This compensation can make the eyelid or brow appear normal when the forehead muscle is active (eg, when raising the eyebrows) but may result in a lower eyelid position when the frontalis muscle is relaxed. Careful consideration should be given to the injection points and depth. Injections in the glabellar region should be superficial so as to avoid deeper penetration of neurotoxin into the inferior frontalis.

Vascular occlusion
Filler-induced vascular occlusion is a rare but potentially serious complication that can occur during dermal filler procedures. It involves the inadvertent injection of filler material into or near a blood vessel, leading to blockage and impaired blood flow, which can result in tissue damage and necrosis. To avoid this complication, it is imperative for physicians to follow meticulous injection techniques, including aspiration before injecting, to confirm that no blood vessels are inadvertently punctured. Moreover, a thorough understanding of facial anatomy, including the location of major blood vessels, is essential. In case of any suspicion of vascular occlusion, immediate intervention is crucial. Prompt administration of hyaluronidase and massage of the affected area can help dissolve HA-based fillers and restore blood flow. Proper education, training, and ongoing monitoring of patients can contribute to the safe and effective use of dermal fillers, minimizing the risk of vascular occlusion.

Tyndall effect
The Tyndall effect is an optical phenomenon that can occur when dermal fillers, particularly HA-based ones, are injected too superficially into the skin. It results in a bluish or grayish

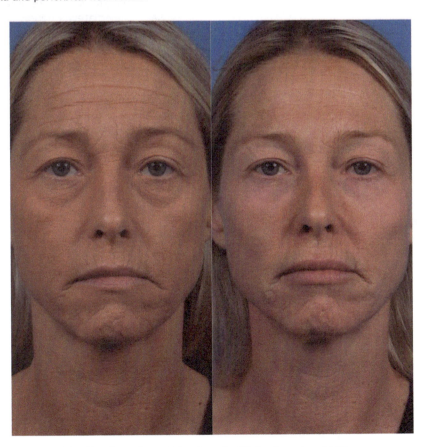

Fig. 7 2 weeks post-treatment with hyaluronic acid filler.

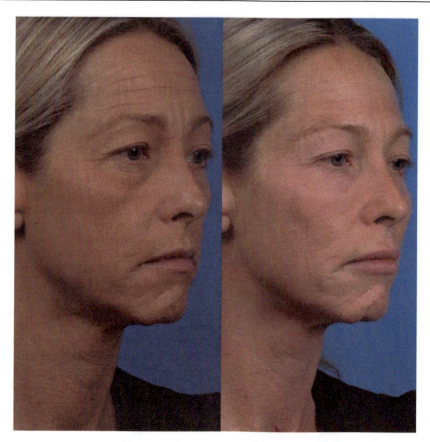

Fig. 8 2 weeks post-treatment with hyaluronic acid filler.

discoloration of the skin at the injection site due to the scattering of light by the filler material. To avoid the Tyndall effect, physicians should ensure proper placement of fillers at an adequate depth within the dermal layers, avoiding the superficial layers where light scattering is more likely. This requires a keen understanding of facial anatomy and precise injection techniques.

"Pearls and pitfalls"

As with any surgery or procedure, patient selection is the first step in ensuring a satisfactory outcome. It is important to distinguish between patients who are good candidates for injectables and those who may be better suited with surgery.

An important component of patient satisfaction is managing expectations. Patients should be made aware that the results from injectables are temporary and typically not as profound as the results that can be achieved with surgery.

Immediate postoperative care
Dermal filler
- Advise the patient not to massage injection sites.
- Advise the patient to ice injection sites.

Botulinum toxin type A
- Advise the patient not to massage injection sites.
- Advise the patient to refrain from exercising and laying supine for 4 hours.

Rehabilitation and recovery

Dermal fillers and neurotoxins have virtually no downtime. Patients should be advised to limit activity for the remainder of the day following the procedure. The effects of dermal fillers can be seen immediately whereas neurotoxins can take anywhere from 3 to 14 days to become active.

Summary

With proper patient selection, injectables in the form of neurotoxins and dermal fillers can safely and predictably be used to rejuvenate the periorbital region. Neurotoxins can be used to elevate the brows and improve periorbital rhytids. Dermal fillers can be used to camouflage tear trough deformity and improve midface volume.

Disclosure

No commercial or financial conflicts of interest or any funding sources.

Suggested reading list

Trinh LN, Grond SE, Gupta A. Dermal fillers for Tear Trough rejuvenation: a systematic review. Facial Plast Surg 2022;38(3):228–39.

Naik MN. Hills and valleys: understanding the under-eye. J Cutan Aesthet Surg 2016;9(2):61–4.

Finn JC, Cox SE. Fillers in the periorbital complex. Facial Plastic Surgery Clinics of North America 2007;15(1):123–32.

Mannino M, Lupi E, Sara B, et al. Vascular complications with necrotic lesions following filler injections: literature systematic review. Journal of Stomatology, Oral and Maxillofacial Surgery 2023: 101499.

Sungat KG, Arisa O. Perioral rejuvenation in aesthetics: review and debate. Clin Dermatol 2022;40(3):265–73.

Ramesh S. Treatment of glabellar frown lines with c. botulinum-a exotoxin. in: foundational papers in oculoplastics. Cham: Springer; 2022.

Lamb J. Volume rejuvenation of the face. Mo Med 2010;107(3): 198–202.

Omran D, Tomi S, Abdulhafid A, et al. Expert opinion on non-surgical eyebrow lifting and shaping procedures. Cosmetics 2022;9(6): 116.

Smith S, , et alMassey BL, Hall MB, et al. A prospective open-label study for treatment of infraorbital hollows using a volumizing hyaluronic acid filler. Facial Plast Surg 2023. https://doi.org/10.1055/a-2102-4796.

Complications of Injectables

Bang Quach, MD, DMD[a,*], Ross A. Clevens, MD[b]

KEYWORDS

- Neuromodulator • Eyelid ptosis • Brow ptosis • Dermal filler • Hyaluronic acid • Hyaluronidase • Vascular injection • Skin necrosis

KEY POINTS

- Understand pertinent facial anatomy prior to the administration of neuromodulators and dermal fillers.
- It is important to undertreat as more can always be added at subsequent follow up appointment.
- Be able to recognize early signs and symptoms of vascular occlusion of dermal fillers.
- Understand the recommended standard dosage of hyaluronidase for addressing vascular occlusion and determining treatment endpoints.

Introduction

In recent years, the demand for non-surgical esthetic procedures has been steadily rising. According to Aesthetic Surgery Report (2022), this category accounts for 28% of the total revenue of $11.8 billion.[1] Neuromodulators, skin treatments, and dermal fillers yield almost 80% of the revenue. They are the preferred choice for individuals seeking to rejuvenate their appearance, reduce signs of aging, and enhance their confidence. What sets neuromodulators and dermal fillers apart from their surgical counterpart is their ability to deliver remarkable results with minimal downtime. Nevertheless, it is important to recognize that even though minimally invasive techniques have brought significant changes to cosmetic medicine and surgery, they are not without their complexities and potential complications.

Complications of neuromodulators

There are currently 5 Food and Drug Administration-approved neuromodulators for facial rejuvenation in the United States. These include Botox (onabotulinumtoxinA), Dysport (abobotulinumtoxinA), Xeomin (incobotulinumtoxinA), Jeuveau (botulinum toxin type A), and Daxxify (daxibotulinumtoxinA-lanm) which basically are all injectables involving botulinum toxin. The difference is in their formulations.

Neuromodulators work by blocking the presynaptic release of the neurotransmitter acetylcholine at the neuromuscular junction, thereby inducing partial paralysis and atrophy of the muscle fibers. Based on this mechanism of action, selective delivery of the toxin to specific facial muscles could help soften fine lines and wrinkles. Therefore, it is imperative for the injector to fully understand the intricacies of facial anatomy and the required dosage to optimize treatments and to avoid unwanted complications.

Incidence of complications

Based on a review of 9398 botulinum toxin treatments, the most common adverse events are headache (5.38%) followed by nasopharyngitis (3.08%), and hypersensitivity reaction (2.90%).[2]

Headache/pain at injection site

Headache could be explained by the injected location of the procedure itself, with underlying cause of periosteal or intramuscular irritation, hematoma, and muscle spasm. The duration of such episode is short and temporary.

Hypersensitivity reactions

Allergic and hypersensitivity reactions although uncommon, have been reported. Transient localized cutaneous reactions, such as diffuse acneiform eruption of the forehead, are reported. Incidents of severe systemic allergy with generalized itching to anaphylaxis are rare.[3,4] Regardless of the severity of the reactions, the type of the hypersensitivity reactions needs to be examined to determine whether it is a type I or type IV, or pseudo-allergy reactions. Remember to rule out whether the disinfectants used could be a culprit in causing the event.

Local injection reactions

Edema, bruising, pain, ecchymosis, and discomfort only account for less than 1% based on the systematic review.[2] In our practice, the incidence of bruising is almost non-existence with the employment of 32-gauge needles, superficial injections, and direct avoidance of visible vessels under the surface of the skin. To further minimize the risk of bruising and patient discomfort, the needle is changed frequently. Patients remain in the office after injection with an ice pack in place for 5 to 10 minutes after their procedure.

Undertreatment and overtreatment

When patients seek neuromodulators for facial wrinkles, it is crucial to assess their treatment history, including prior neurotoxin injections, treated areas, dosages, and satisfaction. For Botox-naïve individuals, conservative treatment is often recommended, with results visible within 24 hours but

---

[a] Facial Plastic & Reconstructive Surgery, 707 West Eau Gallie Boulevard, Melbourne, FL 32935, USA
[b] 707 West Eau Gallie Boulevard, Melbourne, FL 32935, USA
* Corresponding author. 707 West Eau Gallie Boulevard, Melbourne, FL 32935.
E-mail address: phibang2006@gmail.com

optimal outcomes appearing up to 2 weeks post-injection. Follow-up visits ensure patients are satisfied even if touch-ups are not necessary.

Although a minority, some patients request the "frozen" look. It can be a challenge to find this balance to avoid overtreating the region. It is important to recognize that some patients are 'frontalis dependent.' They unconsciously hyper-animate and elevate their brows in order to alleviate brow ptosis or excessive upper eyelid dermatochalasis. In such patients, complete paralysis of the frontalis can appear to worsen this condition as patients can no longer activate the lower portion of the frontalis to lift the brows, which in turn lift the eyelids. They tend to complain that their brows feel heavy, "sleepy", and appear tired.

Brow and eyelid ptosis

Ptosis could be iatrogenic and due to over injection of neuromodulators, trauma, aging, and developmental or genetic abnormalities. In the aging population, droopy brows, and eyelids are often observed. Surgical options are available to address these concerns such as brow lift and blepharoplasty. However, some patients do not want the down time and seek non-surgical options.

It is important to conceptualize that neuromodulators may be used to selectively weaken the antagonizing elevators and depressor of the brow. By weakening the depressors of the brow such as the corrugator, depressor supercilii, and the lateral portion of the orbicularis oculi, the brows can moderately be lifted with neurotoxin application. This is a result of altering the balance of the antagonistic musculature of the brow. On average, patients receive the recommended dosage in the glabellar region of 20 to 24 units in women and 24 to 32 units in men, 2 to 4 units in the lateral-superior portion of the orbicularis oculi, and 4 to 12 units in the lateral portion of the orbicularis oculi, 1 cm lateral from the lateral orbital rim as shown in Fig. 1. However, if the injector is not aware of the anatomic landmarks, ptosis of both the brow and eyelid can occur as shown in Figs. 2 and 3, leading to visual field disturbance.

Managements of brow and eyelid ptosis are often challenging as there are no effective and immediate reversal agents for neuromodulators. It is of paramount importance to prevent these complications from occurring with proper dosing and placement of neurotoxin.

Eyelid ptosis occurs when the injected neurotoxin diffuses through the orbital septum and reaches the levator palpebrae superioris, the elevator the upper lid. There are key anatomic landmarks to in this region. When injecting the lateral corrugator muscle, stay medial to the mid-pupillary line and be superficial, just right under the skin, as shown in Fig. 1. If the depth passes through the orbicularis oculi, there is potential for the toxin to pass through the orbital septum into the posterior lamellae, potentially leading to blepharoptosis.

Blepharoptosis can also be explained by variations in the exit path of the supraorbital pedicles. One is through the supraorbital foramen and the other is through the supraorbital notch. For individuals with a more superior supraorbital foramen, this can be a shorter pathway for the toxin to spread into the orbit as shown in Fig. 4.[5] This can be alleviated by placing the thumb over the supraorbital notch and the injection needle pointing in the superior and lateral direction.

Some authors suggest diluting Botox with 1 mL of normal saline per 100 units yields a more concentrated neurotoxin solution that reduces the risk of toxin diffusion. The lesser volume afforded by this more concentrated dilution can help prevent unwanted diffusion through the supraorbital foramen/notch or into the levator palpebrae superioris if the depth of the injection is too deep. Nevertheless, the injectors need to be extremely precise in delivering the botulinum toxin to have the desired outcome. As a result of this, it is more common to dilute 100 units of Botox with 2.5 cc of normal saline to achieve a balance between precision and diffusion.

Treatment of eyelid ptosis

Several medical management options are available. The ophthalmic drops include oxymetazoline HCl 0.1% (Upneeq), apraclonidine 0.5% (Iopidine), and naphazoline and pheniramine (Naphcon A, available over-the-counter). They are adrenergic agonist agents that targets both alpha-1 and alpha-2 receptors. In addition to the levator palpebrae superioris muscle, which is the main upper lid elevator, Müller's muscle also assists in upper lid elevation. It is comprised of smooth muscle fibers of the sympathetic nervous system. By activating the adrenergic receptors of the Müller's muscle, eyelid ptosis can be ameliorated.

Brimonidine gel 0.33%, an adrenergic agonist, can also be used if patients cannot tolerate ophthalmic drops. It is applied over the skin of the upper eyelid and seems to have much lower side effects profile than the alternatives. Its effect however tends to be short-lived.[6,7]

Anticholinesterases are also an option if patients have a history of local allergy with alpha adrenergic ophthalmic drops. Improvement can be seen within 30 minutes at a 60 mg per os dose of pyridostigmine, effect lasts about 6 to 8 hours.[8]

Transdermal botulinum toxin injection in the pretarsal region to target the orbicularis oculi is another alternative.[9,10] Approximately 2 to 3 units 2 mm above the lash line. Improvement in minimal residual disease is observed between the 6 to 12 weeks mark. This method is technique sensitive. Thus, it is

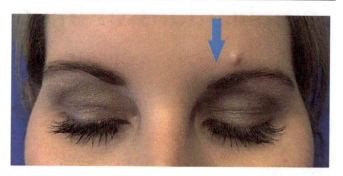

Fig. 2 Left brow ptosis after Botox treatment. Note the medial and middle portions of the left compared to the right brow.

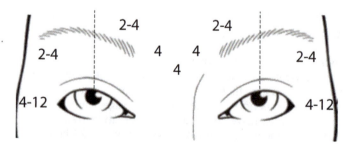

Fig. 1 Illustrative diagram for the typical dosage of Botox for the treatment of brow ptosis. Note that these dosages are starting point.

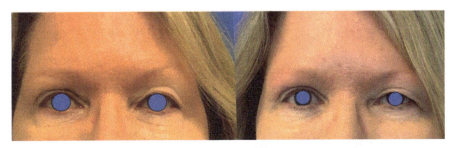

Fig. 3 53-year-old female presented for treatment of left eyelid ptosis. She received the recommended dosage of Botox of 20 units for the glabella region, and 8 units each at 1 cm lateral to the lateral canthus and 2 units each at the tail of the brows. On the right, patient followed up 2 weeks after with sign of blepharoptosis of the left eye.

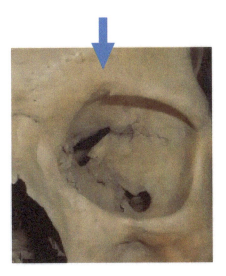 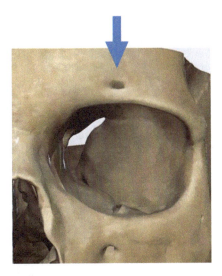

Fig. 4 Comparison between the supraorbital notch (left) and the supraorbital foramen (right). Their locations can serve as retrograde pathway for diffusion of toxin, especially the superiorly placed foramen.

Table 1 Treatment of Eyelid Ptosis, this table lists the currently available medical management of acquired blepharoptosis

Treatment of eyelid ptosis		
Drug	Mechanism of Action	Suggested Dosage
Oxymetazoline HCl 0.1% (Upneeq)	α-adrenergic agonist, stimulation of the Müller's muscle	1 drop up to 2 times per day
Apraclonidine 0.5% (Iopidine)		1–2 drops up to 2–3 times per day
Naphazoline and pheniramine (Naphcon A)		1–2 drops up to 2–3 times per day *available over-the-counter*
Brimonidine Gel 0.33%		0.2 mg applied over the upper lid. Effect lasts up to 2 hour
Pyridostigmine Tablet	acetylcholinesterase inhibitor	60 mg PO up to 3 times per day for 2–3 wk. Effect lasts 6–8 hour per dose
Botox (onabotulinumtoxinA)	partially paralyzes a portion of the orbicularis oculi to aid in lid elevation	2–3 units of Botox in the pretarsal region 2 mm above the lash line

critical to understand that blepharoptosis can worsen if the toxin diffuses into the orbital septum. A more concentrated dilution is ideal in this scenario (Table 1) (Figs. 5 and 6).

Complications of dermal fillers

Dermal fillers are among the most popular non-surgical solutions for restoring lost volume, softening wrinkles, and enhancing facial contours. There are a multitude of dermal fillers in the market, with each one boasting distinct compositions and specific areas of application. They can be grouped in the non-permanent and permanent categories. The non-permanent group include calcium hydroxyapatite (Radiesse), poly-L-lactic-acid (Sculptra), hyaluronic acid (Restylane, Juvéderm), and collagen. The permanent group includes silicones, polyalkylimides, polyacrylamides, and polymethylmethacrylate (Bellafill, indicated for smile lines).]

The concept of dermal fillers appears to be very simplistic, injecting into areas where volume is deficient. Nevertheless, it

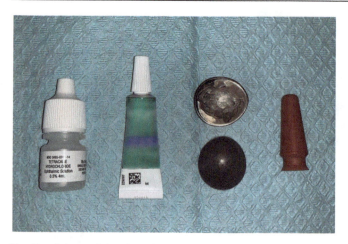

Fig. 5 Prior to injection of Botox in the pretarsal region, 1 to 2 drops of 0.5% of Tetracaine HCl is administered. Then, corneal shield with lubricant eye ointment is placed over patient's affected eye. (*From*: https://systane.myalcon.com/products/systane-nighttime/.)

is crucial to approach dermal fillers with extreme care, as complications, though infrequent, can occur. These potential issues encompass temporary swelling, bruising, infection, or localized lumps at the injection sites. In rarer instances, more severe complications, such as infection or vascular occlusion, may arise. To minimize these risks, it is paramount to understand the compositions and management for each type of filler that you provide for your patients.

Statistics

According to the American Society of Plastic Surgeons (2020), 3.4 million soft-tissue fillers procedures were administered, including both non-permanent and permanent fillers. The complication rates between these 2 groups greatly differ from each other.

From a group of 503 patients who received permanent fillers, 64.61% of patients experienced complications, with onset of symptoms occurred between 1 to 5 years (39.2%), less than 1 year (17.3%), followed by 6 to 10 years (12.61%).[11] The most common symptoms are lumps (64.6%), depression (58%), leathery skin changes (32.2%), granuloma formation (19.1%), and migration and translocation (4.2%). There are no established protocols for the treatment of permanent filler complications. Techniques ranging from disrupting the filler with subcision and transection, surgical removal, liposuction and ultrasound-guided removal, and the injection of triamcinolone or 5-Fluorouracil have been suggested. Due to the wide variability in onset and the types of symptoms present, the most effective means of averting complications associated with permanent fillers may entail refraining from undergoing such treatments altogether.

In contrast, non-permanent fillers are associated with different subset of complications. Although infrequent, they can be severe or permanent, including skin necrosis, vision loss, blepharoptosis, decreased visual acuity, ophthalmoplegia, or encephalitis have been reported. Local edema, skin erythema, headache, and local infection were most common.[12]

Bruising

There is an increase in vascularity along the perioral and lip regions. Bruising and hematoma may occur when multiple injections are administered, especially for lip augmentation. The introduction of the cannula technique, however, has heralded a noteworthy reduction in the incidence of bruising and hematoma[13–19]. Patients now undergo a single precise entry point on each side, typically utilizing a needle of 2 to 3 gauges larger than the canula. This refinement has not only enhanced patient comfort but also witnessed an improved tolerance toward the procedure. Fig. 7 later demonstrates 1 way to perform lip augmentation and the nasolabial fold regions.

Temporary edema

Edema, a temporary inflammatory response, occurs more frequently when bruising is observed at the injection site. In the context of lip augmentation, especially when employing higher-concentration hyaluronic acid fillers like Juvéderm Ultra XC and Ultra Plus XC, lip edema frequently emerges

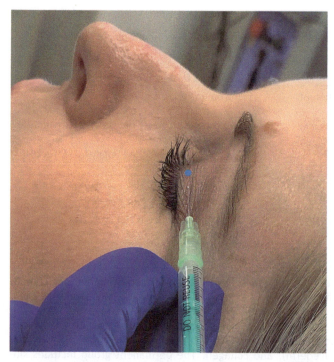

Fig. 6 After placement of corneal shield, the needle is injected from the lateral to medial approach, tangential to the curvature of the lid and 2 mm above the last line. Important to remain superficial to the orbicularis oculi.

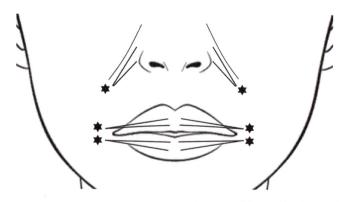

Fig. 7 Diagram illustrating the use of entry point for each side (star mark), using a needle 2 to 3 gauge larger than the canula to dilate the skin opening for easy insertion of the canula. Mild pressure is often required to go through the full half-length of the lip due to fibrous septations.

Table 2 Management of non-permanent filler complications

Adverse events	Onset	Suggested protocol
Tyndall Effect	Immediate	• Tear-trough region — inject 20–50 units of hyaluronidase with gentle massage • Lower face — puncture at the height of the concerned area with a 20-gauge needle, then attempt to express the filler with digital pressure
Contour Irregularities	Immediate	• Firm massage immediately after injection • Perioral region - apply pressure with second finger intraoral and thumb on skin in a circular motion • Advise patient to continue massaging at home
Granuloma	Months	• Triamcinolone 40 mg/ml mixed with 5-fluorouracil in a 1:1 ratio monthly (adjust dosage based on response) • Oral methylprednisolone 50 mg/day for 4 wk[22] • Oral antibiotics (clindamycin 300 mg bid and ciprofloxacin 500 mg tid) for 4 wk[22]

Pustules, vesicles, and abscesses	1–3 d	• Daily local wound care
		• Incision & drainage with abscess formations
		• Daily skin debridement with skin necrosis
		• Oral antibiotics
		    Ciprofloxacin 500 mg bid for 10–14 d
		    If allergic → Levofloxacin 750 mg daily for 10–14 d*
		    Bactrim 800 mg/160 mg bid for 10–14 d
		    If allergic → Doxycycline 100 mg bid for 10–14 d
		    * Cross-reactivity between different generations of fluoroquinolones is uncommon, ranging between 2%–14%[23] Be cautious if hypersensitivity reactions include anaphylaxis

Delayed Hypersensitivity	Weeks to months	Presents as erythema surrounding the treated area • Ciprofloxacin 500 mg bid for 10–14 d or Levofloxacin 750 mg daily for 10–14 d and up to 6 wk • Alternatively, clarithromycin or azithromycin can be used * Avoid steroids and NSAIDS to decrease risk of biofilm formation
Vascular Occlusion	Immediate	Symptoms start with blanching of skin with pain, followed by livedo reticularis at day 1–2, pustules formation around day 3, coagulation of skin and ultimately skin necrosis (days after) • Massage the area and apply warm compress • Mark the area of skin erythema and take photograph • Inject 500–1500 units of hyaluronidase into the marked area of concerns with needle or canula A starting dose of 500 units per area is recommended (lip, nose, forehead). 1000 units if lip and nose are involved. • Reassess capillary refill time and skin color improvement Compare with unaffected side for baseline • Repeat hourly until resolution of symptoms • Close follow up and document with photographs • Consider oral antibiotics if skin discoloration and necrosis

Adapted from: Murray G, Convery C, Walker L, Davies E. Guideline for the Management of Hyaluronic Acid Filler-induced Vascular Occlusion. J Clin Aesthet Dermatol. 2021 May;14(5):E61-E69.

within 1 to 2 days post-injection, potentially persisting for up to 7 to 10 days. Patients, understandably, often express concerns and a desire for filler dissolution. Therefore, it is crucial to make sure patients apprehend the course. It is recommended to avoid modifying filler for at least the first 10 to 14 days after the proper placement of filler. This allows sufficient time for swelling and bruising to resolve fully before evaluating the outcome.

Infection

Infections account for approximately 15% of the rate of transient complications of non-permanent filler.[12] Pustules, vesicles, and abscesses were observed. The onset of symptoms typically starts between 1 to 3 days after the treatment. Management involves daily local wound care, incision and drainage, wound debridement if indicated, and oral antibiotics. A standard regime comprises of ciprofloxacin 500 mg twice daily for 10 to 14 days, and also considers doxycycline 100 mg twice daily or sulfamethoxazole/trimethoprim at 800 mg/160 mg twice daily if methicillin-resistant *Staphylococcus aureus* is suspected.[20,21] It is important to practice aseptic technique before administering treatment. Refer to Table 2 to access the comprehensive management protocol.[22,23]

Individuals with a prior history of herpetic outbreaks in the perioral region should be prescribed a prophylactic regimen of Valtrex at a dosage of 500 mg twice per day, commencing 3 days before the planned injection and continuing for a duration of 7 days following the procedure.

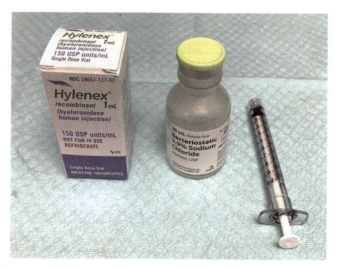

Fig. 8 Hylenex (human recombinant hyaluronidase) comes in a 1 mL vial. Diluting it with 2 mL of normal saline provides 50 units per mL mixture. Hylenex is recommended to be stored between 2 to 8C. (*From*: https://dailymed.nlm.nih.gov/dailymed/fda/fdaDrugXsl.cfm?setid=c3f1db01-58bf-2226-e053-2a95a90a8b33&type=display#:~:text=HYLENEX%20recombinant%20is%20indicated%20as,fluid%20administration%20for%20achieving%20hydration.&text=HYLENEX%20recombinant%20is%20indicated%20as%20an%20adjuvant%20to%20increase%20the,absorption%20of%20other%20injected%20drugs.)

Depth of injection

Tyndall effect arises when light shines through a colloidal mixture, a medium containing microscopically suspended particles, yielding a bluish discoloration due to the refraction of light. This often occurs with superficial injections of hyaluronic acid filler and more so in the thin-skinned area such as the tear-trough region. When the discoloration is faint, it can be mistaken for a bruise. Patient can be observed for 2 weeks if bruising is suspected. If there is no improvement or resolution, the hyaluronic acid filler can be dissolved with hyaluronidase to alleviate the bluish tinge of the Tyndall effect.

Hyaluronidase

Hyaluronidase is an enzyme that causes the degradation of both natural and crosslinked hyaluronic acid dermal fillers. The literature suggests 5 units of hyaluronidase recommended per 0.1 mL of 20 mg/mL hyaluronic acid filler. Some other studies suggest up to 30 units. Due to the wide range of suggested dosages, it is recommended to titrate to effect as the injected doses vastly differ from one region to another, as well as how much of the dermal filler we want to dissolve. Oftentimes, complete dissolution of filler is not necessary. Instead, as noted, hyaluronidase may be titrated to shape or mold the previously placed filler into a more desirable result. In cases of Hylenex (a human recombinant hyaluronidase) which comes in a 1 mL vial containing 150 units. The Aesthetic Complication Expert group[14] recommends a dilution in 1:2 ratio with either sterile water or saline, yielding a total of 3 mL. Some authors recommend diluting with local anesthetic to aid in patients' comfort. However, changing the pH of the constituents can alter the properly of the enzyme (Fig. 8).

Contour irregularities

Lumping of dermal filler occurs when too much filler is injected into a single site resulting in an unwanted palpable of visible accumulation of filler. Firm massage immediately after administering the filler is as important as the precise location of the injection. This is generally true regarding hyaluronic filler. Other dermal fillers, such as Sculptra, which is composed of poly-L-lactic-acid, works within the deep dermis to stimulate patients' own tissue to produce collagen. In turn, it enhances volumes, reduces wrinkles, and improves contours. Nodule formation is a late-onset complication of Sculptra. If a 3:1 dilution is used for injection, the occurrence rate is at 1%. The rate drops dramatically to 0.13% for a 5:1 dilution.[13] In addition, they need to be well mixed. Immediately prior to injecting Sculptra, we have the assistants continue the mixing process in the syringe until the injectors are ready. Hence, it is advised to use larger volumes of more dilute well-suspended Sculptra in order to reduce the risk of contour irregularities (Fig. 9).

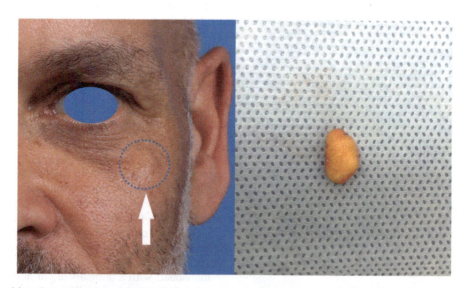

Fig. 9 This 58-year-old male received Sculptra injection into the cheek region to enhance volume. He returned to the clinic after 2 months, complaining of the lump under the skin over his left cheek. After recommending a period of monitoring and massage, the lump did not decrease in size. Thus, patient elected to have it excised. The nodule is shown on the right after removal through a small incision following his natural wrinkle crease.

Vascular occlusion

Vascular occlusion events occur when the target tissue does not receive adequate blood flow to the region. Mechanisms of extravascular compression, vascular spasm, and intravascular embolism were described, with the latter being best supported by evidence.[16] Extravascular compression arises when a large amount of highly viscous filler is injected next to a vessel, especially in areas with low distensibility, such as the nasal tip and nasal dorsum. Hyaluronic acid filler, when injected intravascularly, causes vessel wall inflammation and spasm. Resultant complications do not only occur with the embolus itself, but also as a result of spasm of the surrounding vascular structures. The main areas which have the highest risks of vascular occlusion are the glabellar region, nasolabial fold, nasal tip, and alar triangle.[17]

Signs and symptoms of vascular occlusion could present as immediate or of delayed-onset. Immediate signs and symptoms typically include pain and blanching, followed by reticulated erythema (livedo reticularis) in the distribution of the affected vessel. If this remains untreated, skin necrosis could entail. Filler embolism is another devastating complication associated with intravascular injection, particularly causing visual field deficits or stroke. This phenomenon is explained by retrograde flow proximal to the bifurcation of an artery or through valveless veins of the embolus.

Full resolution of complications can be observed if hyaluronidase is administered once signs and symptoms of impending skin necrosis are recognized early (<2 days).[15] The dosage of hyaluronidase varies and should be based on the amount previously injected and the anatomy of the affected area. Endpoint should be the complete resolutions of symptoms (capillary refill time or skin color has returned to baseline). For simplicity, on an hourly basis, a standard dose of 500 units is administered per area (lip, nose, and forehead) and gentle massage is performed to enhance the distribution of the enzyme.[18] The patient is kept for monitoring 2 to 3 hours after resolution of symptoms and is seen the following day.

Summary

The advent of neuromodulator and dermal fillers has transformed the realm of medical esthetics. They are readily available, provide immediate outcomes, and without downtime. As the annual count of procedures continues to climb, so too does the incidence of complications. Therefore, the significance of thorough training, a deep understanding of facial anatomy, expertise in managing complications, and delivering exceptional patient care cannot be emphasized enough.

Disclosure

Authors have no conflict of interest to declare.

References

[1]. Aesthetic plastic surgery national databank statistic 2022. Aesthetic Society; 2022. In: www.theaestheticsociety.org/media/procedural-statistics.

[2]. Sethi N, Singh S, DeBoulle K, et al. A review of complications due to the use of botulinum toxin a for cosmetic indications. Aesthetic Plast Surg 2021 Jun;45(3):1210–20. Erratum in: Aesthetic Plast Surg. 2022 Feb;46(1):595. PMID: 33051718.

[3]. Haque EK, Darwish YR, Reddick CS. Transient localized cutaneous reaction after onabotulinumtoxinA aesthetic injection. SAVE Proc 2020 Jul 9;33(4):598–600.

[4]. King Rosenfield Lorne, Dean George KardassakisKristen Anne TsiaGrace Stayner. The first case report of a systemic allergy to onabotulinumtoxina (botox) in a healthy patient. Aesthetic Surg J 2014;34(5):766–8.

[5]. Nestor MS, Han H, Gade A, et al. Botulinum toxin–induced blepharoptosis: anatomy, etiology, prevention, and therapeutic options. J Cosmet Dermatol 2021;20:3134–47.

[6]. Wijemanne S, Vijayakumar D, Jankovic J. Apraclonidine in the treatment of ptosis. J Neurol Sci 2017 May 15;376:129–32.

[7]. Alotaibi GF, Alsukait SF, Alsalman HH, et al. Eyelid ptosis following botulinum toxin injection treated with briminodine 0.33% topical gel. JAAD Case Rep 2022;22:96–8.

[8]. Karami M, Taheri A, Mansoori P. Treatment of botulinum toxin-induced eyelid ptosis with anticholinesterases. Dermatol Surg 2007;33(11):1392.

[9]. Taha M, Li Y, Morren J. Oxymetazoline hydrochloride eye-drops as treatment for myasthenia gravis-related ptosis: a description of two cases. Cureus 2023;15(3):e36351.

[10]. Mustak H, Rafaelof M, Goldberg RA, et al. Use of botulinum toxin for the correction of mild ptosis. J Clin Aesthet Dermatol 2018;11(4):49–51.

[11]. Mortada H, Al Saud N, Alaithan B, et al. Complications following permanent filler injection: a prospective cohort study and protocol of management. Plast Reconstr Surg Glob Open 2022;10(11):e4687.

[12]. Oranges CM, Brucato D, Schaefer DJ, et al. Complications of nonpermanent facial fillers: a systematic review. Plast Reconstr Surg Glob Open 2021;9(10):e3851.

[13]. Jin YT, Yu-Fong Chang J, Lang MJ, et al. Cosmetic materials-induced foreign body granuloma at the lower lip. J Dent Sci 2022;17(1):586–8.

[14]. King M, Convery C, Davies E. This month's guideline: the use of hyaluronidase in aesthetic practice (v2.4). J Clin Aesthet Dermatol 2018;11(6):E61–8.

[15]. Sun ZS, Zhu GZ, Wang HB, et al. Clinical outcomes of impending nasal skin necrosis related to nose and nasolabial fold augmentation with hyaluronic acid fillers. Plast Reconstr Surg 2015 Oct;136(4):434e–41e.

[16]. DeLorenzi C. Complications of injectable fillers, part 2: vascular complications. Aesthet Surg J 2014 May 1;34(4):584–600.

[17]. King M, Walker L, Convery C, et al. Management of a vascular occlusion associated with cosmetic injections. J Clin Aesthet Dermatol 2020 Jan;13(1):E53–8.

[18]. DeLorenzi C. New high dose pulsed hyaluronidase protocol for hyaluronic acid filler vascular adverse events. Aesthet Surg J 2017;37(7):814–25.

[19]. Fulton J, Caperton C, Weinkle S, et al. Filler injections with the blunt-tip microcannula. J Drugs Dermatol 2012 Sep;11(9):1098–103.

[20]. Murray G, Convery C, Walker L, et al. Guideline for the management of hyaluronic acid filler-induced vascular occlusion. J Clin Aesthet Dermatol 2021;14(5):E61–9.

[21]. Cadena J, Nair S, Henao-Martinez AF, et al. Dose of trimethoprim-sulfamethoxazole to treat skin and skin structure infections caused by methicillin-resistant Staphylococcus aureus. Antimicrob Agents Chemother 2011 Dec;55(12):5430–2.

[22]. Grass J, Majenka P, Sedlaczek OL, et al. Granulomatous reaction to cosmetic soft tissue filler with late-onset inflammatory response. Acta Derm Venereol 2020 Aug 18;100(15):adv00243.

[23]. Azimi Sara F, Vincent Mainella, Jeffres Meghan N. Immediate hypersensitivity to fluoroquinolones: a cohort assessing cross-reactivity. Open Forum Infect Dis 2022;9(Issue 4):ofac106.

Moving?

Make sure your subscription moves with you!

To notify us of your new address, find your **Clinics Account Number** (located on your mailing label above your name), and contact customer service at:

Email: journalscustomerservice-usa@elsevier.com

800-654-2452 (subscribers in the U.S. & Canada)
314-447-8871 (subscribers outside of the U.S. & Canada)

Fax number: 314-447-8029

**Elsevier Health Sciences Division
Subscription Customer Service
3251 Riverport Lane
Maryland Heights, MO 63043**

*To ensure uninterrupted delivery of your subscription, please notify us at least 4 weeks in advance of move.